A History of the Army Blood Program

HOW LEADERS AND EVENTS SHAPED THE WAY
SOLDIERS RECEIVE LIFESAVING BLOOD

EDWARD A. LINDEKE | COLONEL (RETIRED), MS, US ARMY
Director, Borden Institute

LISA O'BRIEN, PHD
Production Writer-Editor

CHRISTINE GAMBOA, MS, MBA
Creative Director & Production Manager, Fineline Graphics, LLC

The opinions or assertions contained herein are the personal views of the author and are not to be construed as doctrine of the Department of the Army or the Department of Defense. Use of trade or brand names in this publication does not imply endorsement by the Department of Defense.

CERTAIN PARTS OF THIS PUBLICATION PERTAIN TO COPYRIGHT RESTRICTIONS. ALL RIGHTS RESERVED. NO COPYRIGHTED PARTS OF THIS PUBLICATION MAY BE REPRODUCED OR TRANSMITTED IN ANY FORM OR BY ANY MEANS, ELECTRONIC OR MECHANICAL (INCLUDING PHOTOCOPY, RECORDING, OR ANY INFORMATION STORAGE AND RETRIEVAL SYSTEM), WITHOUT PERMISSION IN WRITING FROM THE PUBLISHER OR COPYRIGHT OWNER.

Published by the
OFFICE OF THE SURGEON GENERAL
BORDEN INSTITUTE
US ARMY MEDICAL DEPARTMENT CENTER AND SCHOOL
Fort Sam Houston, Texas
2020

Library of Congress Cataloging-in-Publication Data

Names: Fryar, Ronny A., author. | Borden Institute (U.S.), issuing body.
Title: A history of the Army Blood Program : how leaders and events shaped the way soldiers receive lifesaving blood / Ronny A. Fryar.
Description: Fort Sam Houston, Texas : Borden Institute, US Army Medical Department Center and School, Office of the Surgeon General, 2019. | Includes bibliographical references and index.
Identifiers: LCCN 2018048939 (print) | LCCN 2018050432 (ebook) | ISBN 9780160789861 | ISBN 9780160789878 | ISBN 9780160789885 | ISBN 9780160949395 (alk. paper)
Subjects: | MESH: United States. Army. Blood Program. | Blood Banks—history | Military Medicine—history | Quality Control | History, 21st Century | History, 20th Century | United States
Classification: LCC RM172 (ebook) | LCC RM172 (print) | NLM WH 11 AA1 | DDC 362.17/84—dc23
LC record available at Caution-https://lccn.loc.gov/2018048939

PRINTED IN THE UNITED STATES OF AMERICA

25, 24, 23, 22, 21, 20   5 4 3 2 1

A History of the Army Blood Program

HOW LEADERS AND EVENTS SHAPED THE WAY SOLDIERS RECEIVE LIFESAVING BLOOD

COLONEL RONNY A. FRYAR, MS, MT(ASCP)SBB
MEDICAL SERVICE CORPS, US ARMY (RETIRED)

BORDEN INSTITUTE
US ARMY MEDICAL DEPARTMENT CENTER AND SCHOOL
FORT SAM HOUSTON, TEXAS

Contents

About the Author **vii**
Foreword by The Surgeon General **ix**
Preface **xi**
US Army Blood Program Timeline **xiii**

CHAPTER ONE	The Roots of Army Blood Banking: 1940s and 1950s	**1**
CHAPTER TWO	Blood Program Growth, Standardization, and Coordination: 1960s	**25**
CHAPTER THREE	Commitment to Quality and Safety: 1970s	**51**
CHAPTER FOUR	Review, Refine, and Expand: 1980s	**75**
CHAPTER FIVE	Testing Advances and Quality Assurance: 1990s	**93**
CHAPTER SIX	Modernizing and Addressing New Challenges: 2000s	**117**
CHAPTER SEVEN	Today's Army Blood Program	**167**
CHAPTER EIGHT	The Evolution of Army Blood Supply Units	**181**
Appendix A	Army Blood Blank Fellowship	**201**
Appendix B	Influential People of the Army Blood Program	**211**
Appendix C	Complete List of Army Blood Program Leaders	**221**
Appendix D	US Army Blood Donor Infectious Disease Testing	**225**

Acronyms and Abbreviations **227**
Index **229**

About the Author

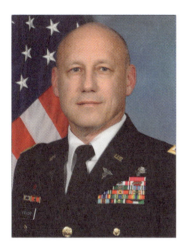

During his Blood Bank Fellowship training in the 1990s, Colonel (Retired) Ronny A. Fryar, MS, MT(ASCP)SBB was required to read Brigadier General Kendrick's book, *Blood Program in World War II*. Each month, his class visited the Armed Services Blood Program Office where Lieutenant Colonel Noel Webster, one of the deputy directors, reviewed blood program operations using examples from Dr. Kendrick's book. Lieutenant Colonel Webster emphasized that learning what our predecessors did would help younger professionals face new challenges in future military operations. The training and mentoring he received during this period laid a strong foundation of respect for history that ultimately resulted in his writing this book.

Colonel Fryar served as the director of the Army Blood Program and as blood program consultant to the surgeon general from 2009 through 2012. During this period he found a copy of Colonel Frank Camp's book *Military Blood Banking 1941-1973: Lessons Learned Applicable to Civil Disasters and Other Considerations*. He was intrigued by many of the historical facts from the Vietnam era and this rekindled his interest in the history of the military blood programs. He also met two other influential military blood bankers, Colonel (Retired) Tony Polk and Colonel (Retired) Jim Spiker, both recipients of the Armed Services Blood Program Lifetime Achievement Award. Colonel Fryar was fascinated by the stories they told, and how each one had a lesson that could be applied to current or future situations.

Colonel Fryar soon realized that it had been nearly 40 years since any history of the Army Blood Program had been published. Since 1973, so much had happened not only in the Army Blood Program, but also in the comprehensive US blood industry. He realized that many of the retired officers held an incredible amount of information and that it was extremely important to capture their stories before they were forgotten. Colonels Polk and Spiker connected Colonel Fryar with many prior and retired Army blood bank officers, and a detailed history began to develop. With assistance from the Army Medical Department museum, Colonel Fryar found more information buried in archives. He also conducted extensive research through the Stimson Library at the Army Medical Department Center and School, US Army Health Readiness Center of Excellence.

Colonel Fryar's goal for this history is to provide current and future Army blood bank officers a source of information that will help them make informed decisions and develop educated strategy as they lead the Army Blood Program into the future. Without any understanding of how the program got to its current point, it will be very difficult for leaders of the Army Blood Program to make the best decisions going forward.

Foreword

Part of being a leader requires one to make good decisions and to envision comprehensive strategic plans. This is not always possible without a knowledge and understanding of the history of an organization or program. From the early roots of the Army's blood program, Major General Douglas Kendrick saw the saw importance of documenting history in his book *The Blood Program in World War II*. It details not only the blood support on the battlefield, but also the decisions that impacted the procurement and delivery of blood to the operational theaters. In 1973, Colonel Frank Camp, Colonel Nicholas Conte, and Lieutenant Colonel Jerry Brewer published *Military Blood Banking 1941-1973: Lessons Learned Applicable to Civil Disasters and Other Considerations*. The primary purpose of this monograph was to apply lessons learned in the military blood program from the end of World War II through the Vietnam War to the medical management of small to medium mass casualties at US civilian medical centers. These leaders knew that it was necessary to pass on experiences and lessons learned to future generations of leaders. However, since 1973, there has not been any published history of the Army Blood Program. The last 40 years have been, perhaps, the most dynamic period in the program's history, with many more outstanding leaders. I am pleased that Colonel Fryar spent the time to capture the tremendous changes and events.

This book weaves together the unique history of the program not only through the usual research of texts and articles, but more importantly through the personal communication with many retired leaders who played critical roles in guiding the program. These individuals provided their own experiences within the program. In addition to supporting various military operations, they oversaw the evolutional changes of the blood supply unit, the implementation of testing for new blood-borne diseases, the birth of the computer age, changes in federal regulatory requirements and accreditation standards, changes in Defense budgets, and research and development of new devices and products—all to better support our military health system.

For anyone who enjoys history, this is a fascinating book to read. I especially encourage the young officers and noncommissioned officers to read and understand how and why the Army Blood Program arrived at this current point in time. You will be the leaders who continue to guide the program in providing high-quality blood products, in an ever-changing environment, to soldiers on future battlefields, and to beneficiaries back home.

RAYMOND S. DINGLE
LIEUTENANT GENERAL, US ARMY
The Surgeon General and
Commanding General, USAMEDCOM

Preface

Throughout over 60 years of history, the Army Blood Program has developed into a leading supplier of blood and blood products for the military. As technology continues to advance; doctrine and requirements continue to evolve; and medical practices, regulations, and the fiscal environment continue to change, the Army Blood Program will undoubtedly adapt to the changing world. However, it will remain dedicated in its mission—providing lifesaving blood.

The Army Blood Program has collected millions of units of blood to support US military members and beneficiaries in peacetime and war. Today, it collects and manufactures hundreds of blood products each day for use in military treatment facilities across the globe. The support of dedicated staff and generous donors within the military community made this possible. Many great leaders have continued to direct the program through countless changes and events. Our predecessors built a strong and successful program. Acknowledging that legacy, present leaders should be reminded of what Colonel Camp noted, "We stand on the shoulders of giants."[1]

COLONEL RONNY A. FRYAR MS, MT(ASCP)SBB
Medical Service Corps, US Army (Retired)

US Army Blood Program Timeline

1940	CPT Captain Douglas B. Kendrick initiates the first blood research program
1942	The Walter Reed General Hospital establishes the first military blood bank
1945	World War II ends
1947	American Association of Blood Banks (AABB) is established
1950	Korean War begins
1952	Department of Defense Directive formally establishes the Armed Forces Blood Donor Program
1953	AABB publishes the first edition of *Technical Methods and Procedures*
1958	The US Army Blood Bank Fellowship (BBF) program is established
1958	AABB publishes the first edition of *Standards for a Blood Bank Transfusion Services*
1962	LTC Lieutenant Colonel Edward O'Shaughnessy, Medical Corps (MC), US Army, is appointed first director of the Military Blood Program Agency
1965	MAJ Major William S. Collins II, introduces a new Styrofoam blood distribution box
1965	Blumberg describes the Australia antigen in serum (which later is referred to as hepatitis-associated antigen, or HAA)
1968	American involvement in the Vietnam War is at its peak
1973	Health Services Command (HSC) is activated on April 26 in San Antonio, Texas
1974	The Army Blood Program begins to be formalized as a program under the newly established Health Services Command (HSC) under the direction of LTC Lieutenant Colonel James Spiker
1975	Brooke Army Medical Center becomes the first Army facility to receive FDA license

1983	Dr. Robert Gallo publishes a paper about the isolation of the virus believed to cause acquired immunodeficiency syndrome (AIDS)
1986	The Army begins HIV human immunodeficiency virus look-back investigations
1988	The *Hepatitis C virus* (the primary agent of Non-A, Non-B hepatitis) is discovered
1989	Operation Just Cause (Panama) takes place
1990	Operations Desert Shield and Desert Storm begin
1991	FDA issues Draft Guidelines for Quality Assurance in Blood Establishments
1992	Operation Restore Hope (Somalia) occurs
1994	Operation Uphold Democracy (Haiti) starts
1995	The FDA publishes the final Guidelines for Quality Assurance in Blood Establishments
1995	The Army Blood Program establishes a civilian quality assurance manager position
1995	Operation Joint Endeavor (Bosnia) starts in December
1996	The Blood Bank Center at Fort Hood becomes the first Army donor center to switch from preservative CPDA-1 (citrate phosphate dextrose adenine) to AS-5 (Optisol, Terumo Corp, Tokyo, Japan), increasing the expiration date of blood units from 35 days to 42 days
1999	Operation Joint Guardian (Kosovo) begins
2001	Operation Enduring Freedom begins
2003	Operation Iraqi Freedom begins
2009	Army Blood Program Quality Assurance Office expands
2010	The Operation Unified Endeavor (Haiti earthquake response) takes place
2011	Walter Reed Army Medical Center closes

REFERENCES

1. Camp FR, Conte N, Brewer JR. *Military Blood Banking 1941–1973–Lessons Learned Applicable to Civil Disasters and Other Considerations*. Fort Knox, KY: US Army Medical Research Laboratory, Blood Bank Center; 1973.

> This book weaves together the unique history of the program not only through the usual research of texts and articles, but more importantly through the personal communication with many retired leaders who played critical roles in guiding the program. These individuals provided their own experiences within the program.
> —NADJA Y. WEST, THE SURGEON GENERAL

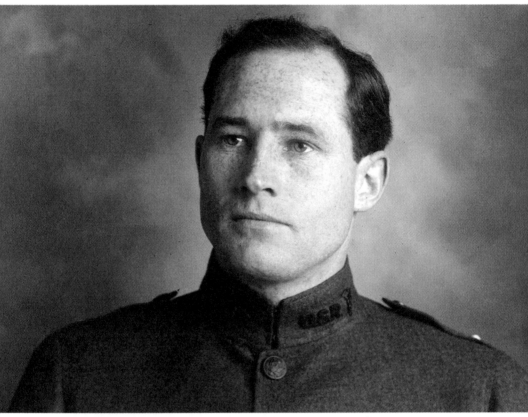

Figure 1-1. Dr. Oswald H. Robertson, Medical Corps, US Reserves. This 5" x 7" glass negative image was taken in 1917, just prior to Robertson's deployment to France. Robertson is wearing his World War I Army uniform. After the war, the British government awarded Robertson the Distinguished Service Order, and in 1958, the American Association of Blood Banks awarded him the Karl Landsteiner Memorial Award. Courtesy of the Rockefeller Archive Center; Record Group 525, Rockefeller University records. ©Rockefeller Archive Center.

CHAPTER ONE

The Roots of Army Blood Banking: 1940s and 1950s

In 1942, the Army was the first service to establish a military blood bank. With roots extending back to World War II, the Army Blood Program has a proud history of providing blood products and services for soldiers, retirees, and their families in both peacetime and war. The establishment of a formal program to oversee blood-collecting facilities, transfusion services, and distribution units has tremendously improved healthcare on the battlefield. During World War II, the case fatality rate (CFR) for the US military was 19.1%. The CFR represents casualties wounded in action who subsequently died, regardless of whether death occurred in a foxhole or in a hospital. In Vietnam, the CFR dropped to 15.8%. By 2006, the CFR for the operations in Iraq and Afghanistan was 6%.[1] This steady decline in the CFR over the decades can be attributed to advancements in military medicine, and the Army Blood Program was a critical component of this success.

WORLD WAR II

Military blood bank efforts can be traced to the work of a young physician, Captain Oswald H. Robertson (Figure 1-1), on the battlefields of World War I, who collected whole blood into glass bottles containing a solution of citrate and dextrose for subsequent transfusion to wounded soldiers.[2] Baxter Laboratories went on to develop the first vacuum glass bottle for whole blood collection and storage in 1939. Baxter's Transfuso-Vac bottle contained sodium citrate that allowed the blood to be stored for 21 days. Before this, blood could be maintained only for a very limited period (hours). Baxter's commercial development realistically allowed quantities of whole blood to be banked for the very first time.[3]

World War II began in September 1939 when Nazi Germany invaded Poland. The United States did not enter into the war until after Japan bombed Pearl Harbor on December 7, 1941. During the 26 months between these dates, President Franklin Roosevelt began to prepare the American people for the high probability of the United States entering the war. At the request of the Department of War, the American Red Cross (ARC) began preparing to collect blood to support the military with whole blood, but focused mostly on providing freeze-dried plasma. On February 4, 1941, the ARC began its National Blood Donor Services with Dr. Charles Drew serving as the medical director. The first ARC regional blood center was in New York. By the end of 1941, 11 ARC donor centers were in operation. Over the next three and a half years, another 24 centers opened.[4]

In 1940, shortly after war broke out in Europe, Captain Douglas B. Kendrick initiated a blood research program at the US Army Medical Field Service School at Carlisle Barracks, Pennsylvania, and served as the program's chief until November 1944. In 1943 Dr. Kendrick was appointed to additionally serve as special representative on blood and plasma transfusions in the Office of The Surgeon General in Washington, DC. In November of that year, the transfusion branch was established at the Office of The Surgeon General. The two entities worked well together: the transfusion branch established policies for the blood and plasma program, while operations were conducted at the Medical Field Service School.[4]

The Walter Reed General Hospital established the first military blood bank in 1942. By 1944, several Army hospitals were able to collect whole blood to meet their own requirements. The European Theater of Operations US Army blood bank collected whole blood from the service members in theater for use in theater. Unfortunately, this effort was not sufficient to meet the growing demand for whole blood; 1,000 pints of type O whole blood were needed daily by 1944. Blood support from the United States was required[5]; however, the military did not have an infrastructure to support these increasing requirements. As a result, the ARC collected most of the blood used to support the military.

The first shipment was flown to Scotland on August 21, 1944. At the time, Alsever's solution[6] proved to be the best preservative solution for blood being shipped overseas. Blood collected in Alsever's solution and continuously refrigerated had a shelf life of 30 days. The next challenge was refrigeration during shipment. In a study, the Army quickly determined that blood left unrefrigerated for 5 days would not produce any transfusion reactions in patients up to 7 or 8 days after collection.[5] A subsequent study looked at the effects on red blood cells if the bottles were refrigerated before a 24-hour flight to the United Kingdom, and then immediately refrigerated upon arrival. The results were that the units could safely be used up to 21 days from collection. However, units were routinely used in 18 days as a precaution.[5]

In an NBC radio address, Major General Paul Hawley, European Theater of Operations chief surgeon, appealed to the American people for increased

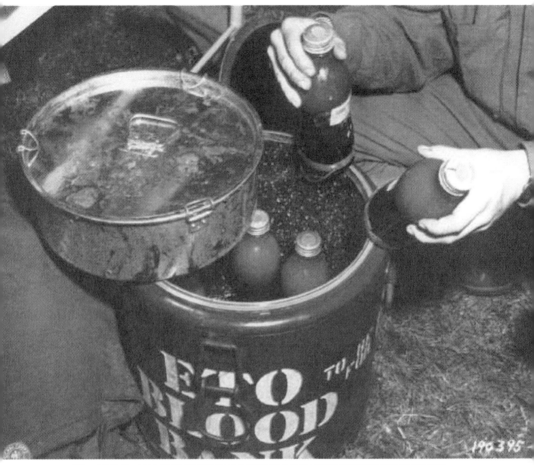

Figure 1-2. During World War II, blood collected in the United States was flown into the European or Pacific theaters using mermite canisters to help maintain the appropriate temperature. Reproduced from: Kendrick DB. *Blood Program in World War II*. Washington, DC: Department of the Army, Office of The Surgeon General; 1964.

donations. He specifically noted that eight centers would collect type O whole blood—five on the East Coast and three on the West Coast. The Army would fly the blood into the European Theater within 24 hours and into the Pacific Theater within 3 days.[7] The first flight to the Pacific Theater occurred in November 1944. Various blood shipping containers that could also be packed with ice came into use in April 1945.[8] Mermite canisters were used as shipping containers to help maintain temperature as the blood was flown overseas (Figure 1-2). Wet ice was placed inside the metal containers and then placed next to the bottle of blood.[4] Other expendable shipping boxes, lined with cork, were also used.[9] Supplies into

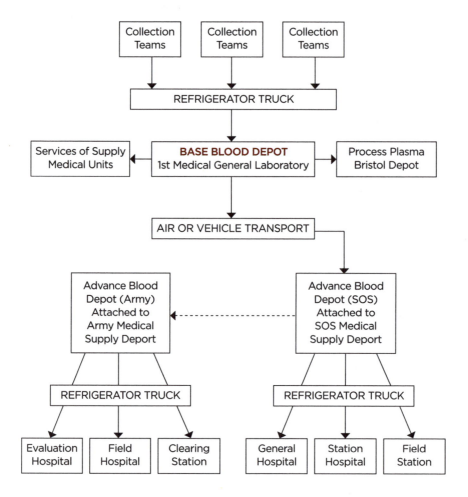

Figure 1-3. Blood distribution in the European Theater of Operations during World War II. Reproduced from: Kendrick DB. *Blood Program in World War II*. Washington, DC: Department of the Army, Office of the Surgeon General; 1964.

the Pacific Theater were also augmented by the Australian Red Cross, transported using heavily insulated wooden shipping boxes.[10]

While efficient procedures to collect, ship, and distribute whole blood for the war effort were being developed and utilized (Figure 1-3), freeze-dried plasma was still the main blood product used on the battlefield. Its use helped restore the blood pressure of injured soldiers, but did nothing to correct hemorrhagic shock. As the war continued, increasing cases of hepatitis led field surgeons to focus more on whole blood.[4]

In 1943, J.F. Loutit and P.L. Mollison developed an acid-citrate-dextrose (ACD) anticoagulant, which preserved red blood cells for 21 days.[4] In addition to preserving blood better, ACD required less volume of solution in each unit of blood compared to Alsever's solution (half whole blood and half Alsever's solution in 1 L bottles). On April 1, 1945, the Army switched to ACD preservative.[4] Using smaller bottles, blood collected in ACD also required less space (600 mL bottles compared to 1 L bottles).[4]

In addition to the actual blood products, crucial durable equipment and expendable supplies were in high demand. During World War II, the military depended heavily on Baxter Laboratories as its commercial source of blood collection products such as glass bottles, flasks, and tubing.[3]

At the end of the war in 1945, the ARC ended its blood program in support of the military. Its blood donor services had collected more than 13 million units of blood during the war. Additionally, Army field hospitals, medical general laboratories, blood transfusion units, and other military units had collected more than 825,000 units. Blood usage during the war was between 0.9 and 1.1 units per casualty.[5]

Between World War II and the Korean War, Army hospitals continued to collect whole blood to meet their own needs.[4] A clinical laboratory officer at Brooke General Hospital, Captain Joseph H. Akeroyd, tested the utilization of plastic blood storage bags from 1947 to 1952. His work eventually led to improved transportation and storage, as well as the ability to separate blood into components—red blood cells and plasma.[11]

KOREAN WAR

In August 1945 the Korean Peninsula became divided along the 38th Parallel when the Soviet Union invaded from the north, and the United States moved in from the south to prevent the Soviet Union from taking over the entire peninsula. Kim Il Sung, the Korean leader in the north, established a communist government. Syngman Rhee established a nationalist government in the south. Both wanted to unify Korea under their particular form of government. On June 25, 1950, the North Korean army crossed the 38th parallel and invaded the south.

With concerns about communism spreading to yet another country, "President [Harry] Truman quickly committed troops to a combined United Nations military effort and named General Douglas McArthur as the Commander."[12]

After the Army Blood Program's formation in World War II, technological advancements during the Korean War led to improvements in the way blood was collected. In the early part of the Korean War, blood was collected and delivered by the 406th Medical General Laboratory in Tokyo, Japan. The laboratory's mission was to control the distribution of blood to hospitals in Japan and mobile hospitals throughout the Pacific Theater of Operations. The 406th sent an escort officer on the overnight flights for shipments to the medical depot in Korea. For receipt of the shipment, the 406th used a chain-of-custody system requiring signatures; the escort officer then returned to Japan on the next flight, according to Colonel (Retired) Jim Spiker's email communication, June 2014. At the same time, type O whole blood was shipped directly from the continental United States to Korea and Japan via air transport. Because of the concern about transfusion reactions, units with high-titer anti-A and anti-B antibodies were given only to type O patients. Low-titer units were given to all other patients. Shipments were taken to the medical supply depots, where blood was stored, and then distributed to hospitals in the combat zone. Initially, mermite canisters were used as shipping containers, but they could hold only a few bottles of blood.[4] As the war progressed, different types of insulated boxes made of plywood or fiberboard were used. These boxes contained a central metal compartment for wet ice, as well as metal racks that held up to 16 bottles of blood, more than what could be shipped in the mermite canisters. The boxes could keep the blood below 10°C for 24 hours. More than 340,000 units of whole blood were flown from the United States to Korea and Japan by the end of the war.[4,5]

The 406th was indispensable in its blood distribution role throughout Korean War. Four years after the ceasefire in February 1957, the 406th medical general laboratory relocated from Tokyo to Camp Zama and the unit eventually became attached to US Army Hospital Camp Zama in January 1966.[13]

In 1951, the Army Medical Graduate School organized a surgical research team and deployed it to Korea and Japan to study the effects of blood transfusions in battle casualties and conduct research on shock. Two members of the team were Lieutenant Colonel William H. Crosby, Medical Corps, and Lieutenant Colonel Joseph H. Akeroyd, Medical Service Corps. Crosby published many articles, and the results of his studies helped set the stage for research eventually conducted at the blood research division of Ft Knox, Kentucky.[4,10]

As the war in Korea intensified, the blood supply from civilian collection agencies in the United States was not sufficient to meet all of the military's blood requirements. As a result, the Armed Forces Blood Donor Program was established

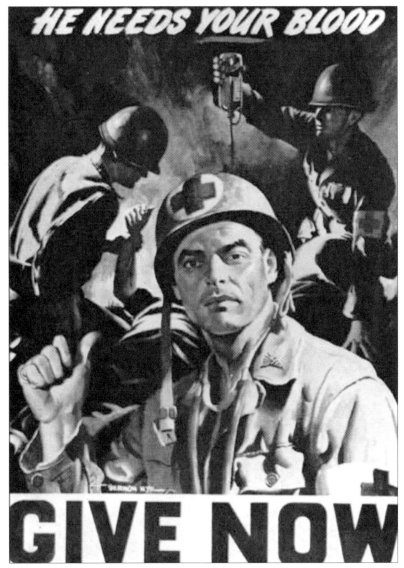

Figure 1-4. The official blood donor recruiting poster of the Armed Forces Blood Donor Program in 1951. Reproduced from: Kendrick, DB. *Blood Program in World War II*. Washington, DC: Department of the Army, Office of The Surgeon General; 1964.

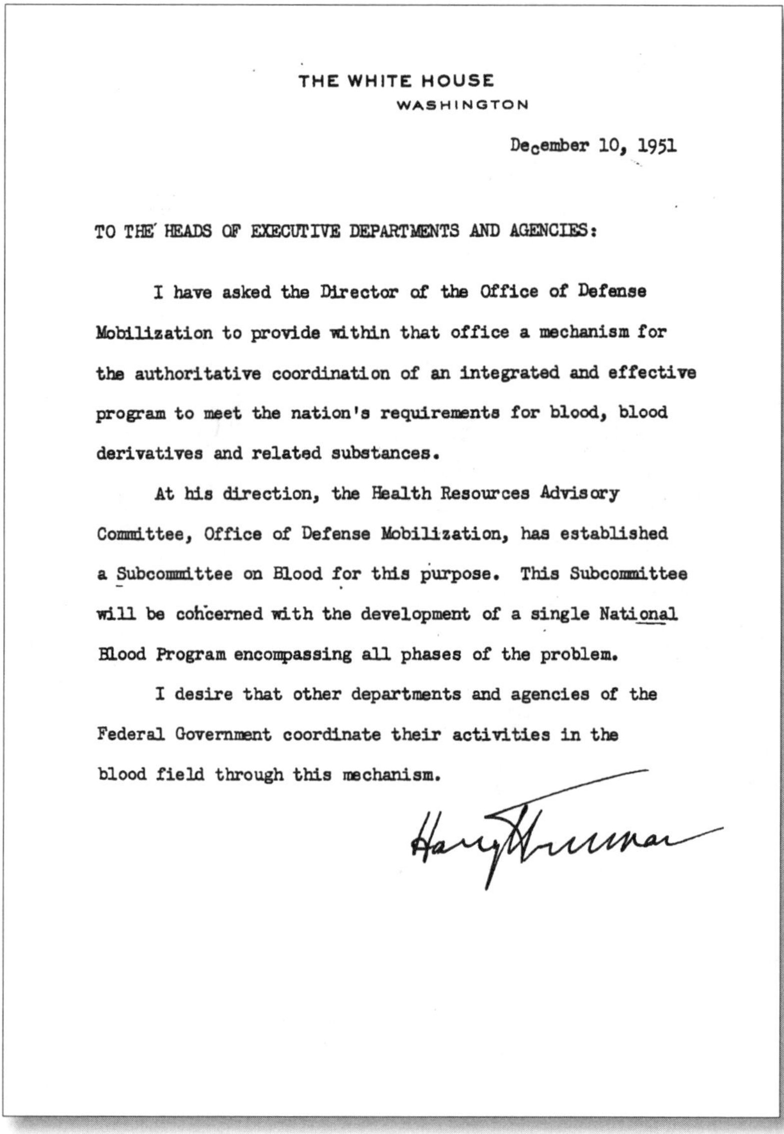

> **THE WHITE HOUSE**
> **WASHINGTON**
>
> December 10, 1951
>
> TO THE HEADS OF EXECUTIVE DEPARTMENTS AND AGENCIES:
>
> I have asked the Director of the Office of Defense Mobilization to provide within that office a mechanism for the authoritative coordination of an integrated and effective program to meet the nation's requirements for blood, blood derivatives and related substances.
>
> At his direction, the Health Resources Advisory Committee, Office of Defense Mobilization, has established a Subcommittee on Blood for this purpose. This Subcommittee will be concerned with the development of a single National Blood Program encompassing all phases of the problem.
>
> I desire that other departments and agencies of the Federal Government coordinate their activities in the blood field through this mechanism.
>
> *Harry Truman*

Exhibit 1-1. President Harry Truman letter to the heads of executive departments and agencies, December 10, 1951. Courtesy of the Truman Presidential Library.

by Department of Defense (DoD) Directive 750.10-1 on August 2, 1951 (Attachment 1-1).[14] The goal of the program was to coordinate the supply efforts from the military, the ARC, and civilian blood banks, and to "persuade civilian and military populations to contribute whole blood in support of the Armed Forces."[14] Figure 1-4 shows the official poster of the Armed Forces Blood Donor Program. In response to the directive, the Army issued Memorandum 1-40-1, Blood Donor Campaign, on November 1, 1951,[15] directing Department of the Army agencies to participate in the Armed Forces Blood Donor Program (Attachment 1-2). It also established the assistant secretary of the Army for manpower and reserve forces as the "chairman of the Army Blood Donor Program" to provide oversight of the donor recruitment effort.

In addition to collecting blood to support the military requirements, a growing concern in America was how to meet the blood needs of civil defense (Figure 1-5). President Truman directed Charles E. Wilson, director of the Office of Defense Mobilization, to develop a mechanism to coordinate the collection and distribution of blood to support the military and civilian hospitals across the United States. Wilson appointed a subcommittee on blood to establish a coordinated program to meet the nation's blood requirements. On December 10, 1951, President Truman sent a letter to the heads of executive departments and agencies requesting that they synchronize blood program collections and distributions through the subcommittee on blood (Exhibit 1-1). The ARC and the DoD requested the Office of Defense Mobilization to assume overall responsibility for the allocation of blood to the DoD and the newly created Federal Civil Defense Administration. The subcommittee, working through the Health Resource Advisory Committee of the Office of Defense Mobilization, developed and issued DoD Directive 6480.1, *National Blood Program*, on July 8, 1952 (Attachment 1-3).[16] Other key principles of the program included establishing national reserves of plasma and its derivatives, prioritizing allocation, and setting up a program to supply "well-trained medical officers in all phases of blood banking and logistics."[4]

The National Blood Program existed until it was replaced by the National Emergency Blood Program on April 10, 1972 (Attachment 1-4),[17] the policies for which are found in the Code of Federal Regulations (CFR), Title 32A, *National Defense*. As a means to ensure available resources in response to a national emergency, the policies establish coordination guidelines for federal agencies. Paragraph 5(b)(2) directs the DoD to restrict military blood donor center activities to military installations only.[12] To ensure minimal impact for civilian communities, military blood teams could only conduct blood drives, collecting blood from donors, on military installations.[12] They were not permitted to conduct drives in the civilian communities as this was viewed as taking donors away from civilian agencies and

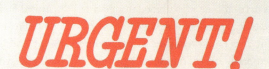

Figure 1-5. A poster from the Department of Defense's blood donor recruitment campaign in support of the newly established Armed Forces Blood Donor Program circa 1951—1952. Reproduced from: US National Library of Medicine Digital Collections. http://resource.nlm.nih.gov/101580733.

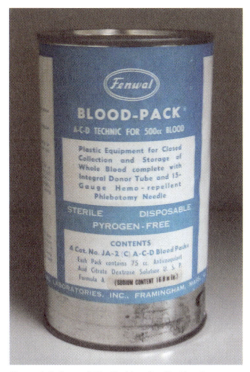

Figure 1-6. Fenwal Plastic blood collection bag sealed in a can, circa 1953. Courtesy of Colonel (Ret) Ronny A. Fryar.

hindering their ability to meet their requirements. Although not specified by the CFR, recruiting and advertising for donors followed the same pattern. Military recruited only on military property. Civilian agencies were to only recruit in the civilian communities.

The National Blood Program directive of 1952 described the national program's coordination efforts (see Attachment 1-3). (Despite aid from the archivist at the Truman Library, a presidential or executive order linked to the National Blood Program, as referenced in other publications, could not be identified.) The presidential order referenced in paragraph 3 of DoD Directive 6480.1 most likely characterizes President Truman's intent ("desire") in the letter of December 10, 1951, as a military order from the commander-in-chief to the DoD. One month after the Korean War armistice was signed, the directive was updated (August 20, 1953) to provide guidance to military commanders, directing military blood collecting centers to provide whole blood to military hospitals, and add clarity of the oversight responsibility for military blood policy to the assistant secretary of defense (health and medical).[18]

During the latter part of the war, Fenwal Laboratories developed and marketed a plastic bag to collect and store blood. Previously, glass bottles had been used exclusively. The bag was designed to contain 500 mL of whole blood using ACD. Each bag was sealed in a can for sterility and could be opened with a key-wind or rotary can opener (Figure 1-6). Although plastic bags could now be used to collect blood, they were not used in the Korean Theater, and it was not until 1957 that military hospitals began using them routinely. However, just as Akeroyd had envisioned earlier, the new bags led to improved transportation and storage as well as easier blood component separation.[4,10] Packed red blood cells were separated by gravity overnight, according to Colonel (Retired) Anthony Polk in his email communication dated January 2011. The transition to plastic blood collection bags also significantly reduced the problem of air embolisms associated with vacuum bottles.[4]

It was difficult to forecast Korean War blood requirements because of the unpredictable casualty rates and lack of documentation about how many units were transfused to patients. Medical leaders looked at historical blood usage rates from the United States and Britain. They studied the transfusion rates at the different Army echelons and the number of transfusions by wound severity. When aggregating the theater and all types of wounds, the average was 4.3 units per casualty.[19] Blood usage per casualty ranged from 1.9 to 5.5 units.[10]

Throughout the Korean War and the remainder of the decade, the Army Blood Program made great strides toward providing a higher-quality blood product to ill or injured soldiers worldwide. The program made advancements in blood storage, collection, and separation that started the progression toward current technologies.

SUMMARY

The destructive military conflicts of the 1940s and 1950s highlighted the importance of blood products in casualty survival. Having blood and plasma on the battlefield allowed for more complex surgeries to be performed, thus improving the survivability from battle-inflicted wounds. The means to provide timely distribution and availability of blood and the processes developed for effective use saved many thousands of lives on and off battlefield. The technological advances made during this period provided a strong foundation for future blood banking successes.

REFERENCES

1. Holcomb JB, Stansbury LG, Champion HR, Wade C, Bellamy RF. Understanding combat casualty care statistics. *J Trauma*. 2006;60:397–401.
2. Hess JR, Schmidt PJ. The first blood banker: Oswald Hope Robertson. *Transfusion*. 2000;40:110–113.
3. Baxter Laboratories website. http://www.baxter.com/about_baxter/company_profile/history.html. Accessed May 31, 2016.
4. Kendrick DB. *Blood Program in World War II*. Washington, DC: Department of the Army; 1964.
5. Kendrick DB Jr, Elliott J, Reichel J Jr, Vaubel EK. Supply of preserved blood to European Theater of Operations. *Bull US Army Med Dept*. January 1945;84:66–67. http://stimson.contentdm.oclc.org/cdm/singleitem/collection/p15290coll6/id/1637/rec/180. Published August 30, 2011. Accessed May 31, 2016.

6. Alsever JB, Ainslic RB. A new method for the preparation of dilute blood plasma and the operation of a complete transfusion service. *N Y State J Med.* 1941;126.
7. Blood transfusion in the reparative management of battle wounds. *Bull US Army Med Dept.* February 1945;85:4–5. http://stimson.contentdm.oclc.org/cdm/singleitem/collection/p15290coll6/id/1659/rec/1. Published September 2, 2011. Accessed December 18, 2014.
8. Whole blood—new refrigeration system. *Bull US Army Med Dept.* June 1945;89:3–4. http://stimson.contentdm.oclc.org/cdm/singleitem/collection/p15290coll6/id/1972/rec/187. Published October 12, 2011. Accessed May 31, 2016.
9. Blood transfusion service. *Bull US Army Med Dept.* December 1946;6:646–649. http://stimson.contentdm.oclc.org/cdm/singleitem/collection/p15290coll6/id/3224/rec/1. Published December 20, 2011. Accessed May 31, 2016.
10. Camp FR, Conte N, Brewer JR. *Military Blood Banking 1941–1973–Lessons Learned Applicable to Civil Disasters and Other Considerations.* Fort Knox, KY: US Army Medical Research Laboratory, Blood Bank Center; 1973.
11. US Department of the Army. *Annual Report of the Surgeon General, United States Army 1972/73–1974/75.* Washington, DC: DA, Office of The Surgeon General; 1975. http://babel.hathitrust.org/cgi/pt?q1=blood;id=uc1.b3994054;view=1up;seq=208;num=66;start=1;sz=10;page=search#view=1up;seq=208. Published August 9, 2013. Accessed May 31, 2016.
12. US National Archives and Records Administration. Teaching with documents: The United States enters the Korean conflict. http://www.archives.gov/education/lessons/korean-conflict/. Accessed May 31, 2016.
13. US Department of Defense. US Army Medical Command Japan. https://www.usamcja.com/history_usamcj2.htm. Accessed April 14, 2014.
14. US Department of Defense. *The Armed Forces Blood Donor Program.* Washington, DC: DoD; 1951. DoD Directive 750.10.
15. US Department of the Army. *Blood Donor Campaign.* Washington, DC: DA; 1951. Memorandum 1-40-1.
16. US Department of Defense. *National Blood Program.* Washington, DC: DoD; 1952. DoD Directive 6480.1.
17. Defense Mobilization Order 8540.2—policy guidance for a national emergency blood program. *Fed Regist.* 1967;32(73).
18. US Department of the Defense. *National Blood Program* (updated). Washington, DC: DoD; 1953. DoD Directive 6480.1.
19. Steer A, Hullinghorst RL, Mason RP. The blood program in the Korean War. In Crosby WH, ed. *Tools for Resuscitation.* Vol. 2. In: *Battle Casualties in Korea—Studies of the Surgical Research Team.* Washington, DC: US Army Medical Department; 1955. http://history.amedd.army.mil/booksdocs/korea/Vol2-BattleCasualties/vol2bc.html. Updated June 3, 2009. Accessed June 1, 2016.

CANCELLED BY: DODD 6480.1, JULY 8, 1952

2 August 1951
Number 750.10-1

Department of Defense Directive
Washington 25, D.C.

TITLE   750 - MEDICAL AND HEALTH

SUBTITLE   10 - WHOLE BLOOD, DERIVATIVES, SUBSTITUTES

NUMBER   750.10-1
              The Armed Forces Blood Donor Program

1. Department of Defense supplies of dried human blood plasma have been gravely depleted by the demands of the Korean campaign. Its continued availability for military purposes is vital. It is imperative that action be taken to insure that an adequate supply is at all times ready for use. This means that every possible effort must be made to secure whole blood in quantity from all available sources.

2. While the processing capacity for converting whole blood to plasma has been gradually increased, the quantities of blood received from civilian sources is today woefully inadequate, and well below processing capacity. The essential reserve is not being created.

3. Accordingly, the Department of Defense will begin immediately:

    a. A continuous and vigorous campaign, in conjunction with the Red Cross, to persuade the civilian and military population to contribute whole blood to the Armed Forces.

    b. To establish an Armed Forces blood donor program within the framework of the overall campaign, the primary purpose of which shall be to obtain blood from service personnel on military bases within the continental United States. Civilian employees will be invited to participate.

863097

Attachment 1-1.

CANCELLED BY: DODD 6480.1, JULY 8, 1952

2 August 1951
750.10-1

4. The Red Cross has agreed to coordinate the collection of blood, primarily from the civilian population, through its existing facilities, cooperating blood banks, and additional Defense Centers established by the Red Cross with Department of Defense funds. Full cooperation by all echelons of the three Services is urged in convincing the civilian population and military personnel of the vital military necessity of supporting this program.

5. The responsibility for promotion, publicity and public information of this campaign, plus any free or paid advertising, is assigned for direction and programming to the Directorate of Public Information, Office of the Secretary of Defense. It is desired that both headquarters and field public information offices of the Services lend their full and whole-hearted support.

6. The Armed Forces blood donor portion of the overall program will be under the policy guidance of the Armed Forces Medical Policy Council, Office of the Secretary of Defense. Responsibility for general direction and control of this military portion of the overall program, its comprehensive coordination, integration of shipping schedules and quotas to laboratories, necessary reporting procedures, and technical guidance, is assigned to the Directorate of the Armed Services Medical Procurement Agency, Main Navy Building, Washington 25, D. C., to which all local Armed Forces blood donor programs must be submitted for approval prior to actual collection of blood in order to avoid waste. Existing medical facilities and personnel should be used to the greatest possible extent. In addition, when practicable and within reasonable geographical proximity, the Armed Forces blood donor program should be coordinated with the local Red Cross facilities or cooperating blood banks. The urgency and nature of this program require direct communication, which should be authorized. Necessary funds will be made available by the Directorate from the Department of Defense Blood and Blood Derivatives Fund. It is understood that blood collected in connection with the Armed Forces blood donor program becomes government property and will be shipped to designated facilities as prescribed.

Acting Secretary

2

Attachment 1-1. Continued

Memo 1-40-1

MEMORANDUM)
No. 1-40-1   )

DEPARTMENT OF THE ARMY
Washington 25, D. C., 1 November 1951

ADMINISTRATION

BLOOD DONOR CAMPAIGN

	Paragraph
General	1
Responsibility	2
Conduct of campaign	3
Appendix	-

1. **General**. In compliance with Department of Defense directive 750.10-1 (App.), and by direction of the Secretary of the Army, each agency of the Department of the Army will actively participate in the Armed Forces Blood Donor Program now being conducted throughout the Army Establishment.

   a. All qualified military and civilian personnel of the Department of The Army within The Pentagon will be asked to donate blood voluntarily at the Pentagon Blood Donor Center.

   b. Personnel of Department of the Army agencies, housed elsewhere than The Pentagon will be asked to donate blood voluntarily at their respective places of employment and duty, when facilities are provided.

2. **Responsibility**. The Assistant Secretary of the Army (Manpower and Reserve Forces) is the Chairman of the Army Blood Donor Program and exercises a general supervision over this campaign.

   a. The head of each agency of the Department of the Army will be responsible for the conduct of the campaign within his own agency and will designate a Recruiting Officer of field grade, or civilian of grade GS-12 or higher, to recruit and schedule blood donors within the agency. The assistance of personnel who are already engaged in this activity will be fully utilized.

   b. The name, grade, room, and telephone number of each Recruiting Officer will be reported promptly to the Vice Chairman of the Blood Donor Program, Office of the Secretary of the Army, Room 3E 739, Extension 55378.

   c. The Chief of Information will provide a continuing program which will acquaint departmental personnel with the purpose and importance of the campaign, and which will inform the public of its progress and accomplishment.

3. **Conduct of campaign**. The campaign will be conducted within each Department of the Army agency in a manner which will provide a constant and regular number of blood donors each week.

Attachment 1-2.

Memo 1-40-1

   a. Quotas for donors will be assigned to each agency in accordance with the availability of blood collecting facilities. It is important that assigned quotas be fully met in order to insure maximum utilization of these facilities. This will be accomplished by advance planning, in which the head of each agency keeps alternative donors available, to give blood when scheduled donors are unable to appear.

   b. The head of each agency will maintain a record of progress covering each calendar month, which will include the following information:

   (1) The number of personnel, both military and civilian, on duty with the agency.
   (2) The number of donors who have given blood during the calendar month.
   (3) The number of blood donors scheduled for each of the 3 months which follow the current month.

   c. For the purpose of planning and control each agency will establish its own long-range quota of voluntary blood donorship. As a guide, it is felt that each agency's quota should exceed an average of 1 pint of blood a person each year.

   d. The American Red Cross has agreed to provide additional facilities necessary to care for the increased donorship developed by this campaign.

   e. The spirit of friendly competition between individuals, offices, and agencies will help to insure the success of the program and is encouraged.

   (AG 742 (31 Oct 51))

   BY ORDER OF THE SECRETARY OF THE ARMY:

OFFICIAL:
WM. E. BERGIN
Major General, USA
The Adjutant General

J. LAWTON COLLINS
Chief of Staff, United States Army

DISTRIBUTION:
Department of the Army

Attachment 1-2. Continued

Memo 1-40-1

APPENDIX

2 August 1951
Number 750.10-1

Department of Defense Directive
Washington 25, D.C.

TITLE   750 - MEDICAL AND HEALTH

SUBTITLE   10 - WHOLE BLOOD, DERIVATIVES, SUBSTITUTES

NUMBER   750.10-1
The Armed Forces Blood Donor Program

1. Department of Defense supplies of dried human blood plasma have been gravely depleted by the demands of the Korean campaign. Its continued availability for military purposes is vital. It is imperative that action be taken to insure that an adequate supply is at all times ready for use. This means that every possible effort must be made to secure whole blood in quantity from all available sources.

2. While the processing capacity for converting whole blood to plasma has been gradually increased, the quantities of blood received from civilian sources is today woefully inadequate, and well below processing capacity. The essential reserve is not being created.

3. Accordingly, the Department of Defense will begin immediately:

   a. A continuous and vigorous campaign, in conjunction with the Red Cross, to persuade the civilian and military populations to contribute whole blood to the Armed Forces.

   b. To establish an Armed Forces blood donor program within the framework of the overall campaign, the primary purpose of which shall be to obtain blood from service personnel on military bases within the continental United States. Civilian employees will be invited to participate.

Attachment 1-2. Continued

Memo 1-40-1

4. The Red Cross has agreed to coordinate the collection of blood, primarily from the civilian population, through its existing facilities, cooperating blood banks, and additional Defense Centers established by the Red Cross with Department of Defense funds. Full cooperation by all echelons of the three Services is urged in convincing the civilian population and military personnel of the vital military necessity of supporting this program.

5. The responsibility for promotion, publicity and public information of this campaign, plus any free or paid advertising, is assigned for direction and programming to the Directorate of Public Information, Office of the Secretary of Defense. It is desired that both headquarters and field public information offices of the Services lend their full and whole-hearted support.

6. The Armed Forces blood donor portion of the overall program will be under the policy guidance of the Armed Forces Medical Policy Council, Office of the Secretary of Defense. Responsibility for general direction and control of this military portion of the overall program, its comprehensive coordination, integration of shipping schedules and quotas to laboratories, necessary reporting procedures, and technical guidance, is assigned to the Directorate of the Armed Services Medical Procurement Agency, Main Navy Building, Washington 25, D. C., to which all local Armed Forces blood donor programs must be submitted for approval prior to actual collection of blood in order to avoid waste. Existing medical facilities and personnel should be used to the greatest possible extent. In addition, when practicable and within reasonable geographical proximity, the Armed Forces blood donor program should be coordinated with the local Red Cross facilities or cooperating blood banks. The urgency and nature of this program require direct communication, which should be authorized. Necessary funds will be made available by the Directorate from the Department of Defense Blood and Blood Derivatives Fund. It is understood that blood collected in connection with the Armed Forces blood donor program becomes government property and will be shipped to designated facilities as prescribed.

Acting Secretary

Attachment 1-2. Continued

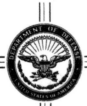

8 July 1952
NUMBER 6480.1

Department of Defense Directive

SUBJECT National Blood Program

Reference: (a) 6480.1, Medical and Health: Whole Blood, Derivatives, Substitutes; The Armed Forces Blood Donor Program, 2 August 1951.

I. **PURPOSE**

The purpose of this directive is to reissue reference (a) to conform with recent developments on the National Blood Program.

II. **CANCELLATION**

Reference (a) is cancelled.

III. **COORDINATING ORGANIZATION FOR NATIONAL BLOOD PROGRAM**

By Presidential order, responsibility for providing a mechanism for the authoritative coordination of an integrated and effective program to meet the nation's requirements for blood, blood derivatives and related substances has been placed within the Office of Defense Mobilization. The Health Resources Advisory Committee, Office of Defense Mobilization, has established a Sub-committee on Blood for this purpose. Activities of the Department of Defense in the blood field will be coordinated with those of other agencies of the government through this mechanism.

IV. **TITLE**

The "Armed Forces Blood Donor Program" will be continued as the Department of Defense interest in the "National Blood Program." The title, "National Blood Program," will be used in public information activities aimed at the recruitment of blood donors in coordination with the American National Red Cross and the Federal Civil Defense Administration through the Office of Defense Mobilization.

Attachment 1-3.

8 July 1952
6480.1

V. NEED

Department of Defense interest in the National Blood Program is two-fold: (1) whole blood and blood plasma are needed for treatment of the wounded on the battlefield and in Service hospitals throughout the world; (2) and blood is needed to continue the build-up of the reserve of plasma ready for any emergency.

VI. ACTION

The Department of Defense will continue:

A. To wage a vigorous campaign, through the Office of Defense Mobilization in coordination with the American Red Cross and Federal Civil Defense Administration, to persuade the civilian and military population to contribute whole blood to the Armed Forces.

B. To operate Armed Forces Blood Donor Centers within the framework of the National Blood Program, the primary purpose of which shall be to obtain blood from service personnel on military bases within the continental United States. Civilian employees will continue to be invited to participate. Civilians of nearby communities may be invited to participate where no other collection facilities for the National Blood Program exist for their use.

VII. COLLECTION COORDINATING AGENCY

The American National Red Cross is designated as the National Blood Program coordinating agency for the collection of blood, primarily from the civilian population, through its existing facilities and cooperating blood banks. Continued full cooperation by all echelons of the three Services is urged in convincing the civilian population and military personnel of the vital military necessity of supporting this program.

VIII. PUBLIC INFORMATION

Policy guidance for the publicity program will be given by a public information steering committee, on which there will be both medical and public information representation from the Department of Defense, the American Red Cross, and the

- 2 -

Attachment 1-3. Continued

8 July 1952
6480.1

Federal Civil Defense Administration, with liaison from the Office of Defense Mobilization. The Department of Defense's share of the responsibility for promotion, publicity and public information of the National Blood Program is assigned to the Director, Office of Public Information, Office of the Secretary of Defense. It is desired that both headquarters and field public information and recruiting offices of the Services continue to lend their full and whole-hearted support. This support includes assignment by the military departments of officer and enlisted military personnel for temporary duty at such times and places as success of the program may require.

IX. The Armed Forces blood donor portion of the overall program continues under the policy guidance of the Armed Forces Medical Policy Council, Office of the Secretary of Defense. Responsibility for general direction and control of this military portion of the overall program, its comprehensive coordination, integration of shipping schedules and quotas to laboratories, necessary reporting procedures, and technical guidance, is assigned to the Directorate of the Armed Services Medical Procurement Agency, Main Navy Building, Washington 25, D.C., to which all local Armed Forces blood donor programs must be submitted for approval prior to actual collection of blood in order to avoid waste. Existing medical facilities and personnel should be used to the greatest possible extent. In addition, when practicable and within reasonable geographical proximity, the Armed Forces blood donor program should be coordinated with the local Red Cross facilities or cooperating blood banks. The urgency and nature of this program require direct communication, which should be authorized. Necessary funds will be made available by the Directorate from the Department of Defense Blood and Blood Derivatives Fund. It is understood that blood collected in connection with the Armed Forces blood donor program becomes government property and will be shipped to designated facilities as prescribed.

William C. Foster
Acting Secretary of Defense

- 3 -

Attachment 1-3. Continued

Title 32A—NATIONAL DEFENSE, APPENDIX

Chapter I—Office of Emergency Planning

[Defense Mobilization Order 8540.2]

DMO 8540.2—POLICY GUIDANCE FOR A NATIONAL EMERGENCY BLOOD PROGRAM

1. *Purpose.* This order prescribes the objectives, policies, and responsibilities of the National Emergency Blood Program.

2. *Cancellation.* The National Blood Program Statement of Basic Principles, dated December 1, 1962, is hereby rescinded.

3. *Background.* Provision of adequate blood and related items and activities to meet basic military, civil defense and civilian needs in an emergency is of recognized national importance. Certain government agencies and civilian blood banking systems have developed programs designed to contribute to this end. Coordination of these programs is essential to achieve maximum effectiveness and to avoid duplication of efforts and conflict of activities.

4. *Objectives.* The National Emergency Blood Program is established to develop, prior to a national emergency, a capability and readiness to make maximum use of available resources to meet the Nation's requirements for blood and related products in any such emergency. Actions directed toward this objective include planning and organization for emergency operations, standardization, and stockpiling of supplies and equipment, training of personnel in blood program techniques, and development of donor appeal measures.

5. *Policy*—(a) *Coordination.* No Federal agency shall duplicate the efforts of any other agency participating in this program except in situations where it is clearly recognized that the task in question cannot be otherwise adequately performed. Further, any such duplicating effort shall not be undertaken without prior agreement among the Federal agencies involved and the Office of Emergency Planning. All other agencies participating in the program are urged to coordinate their efforts with all other participants so as to avoid unnecessary duplication.

(b) *Blood collection activities.* (1) The blood collection activities of Federal agencies shall be administered so as to make maximum, efficient use of available sources while assuring minimum impact on provision of normal blood supplies for the civilian community.

(2) The collection facilities of the Department of Defense shall be limited to Armed Services installations and blood shall be drawn only from military personnel or from civilian personnel on military installations.

(c) *Reserves.* (1) Reserves of blood products, artificial plasma volume expanders and related items shall be established and maintained by the Department of Defense and by the Department of Health, Education, and Welfare.

(2) Blood derivative reserves for the National Emergency Blood Program shall be established by contracting with the civilian suppliers for the collection of blood for this purpose, except that the Department of Defense may utilize blood salvaged from its blood collection program for the purpose of adding to the Department of Defense blood derivative reserve.

(3) Blood or blood derivatives going into the reserves shall be allocated according to military and nonmilitary defense requirements to the Department of Defense and the Department of Health, Education, and Welfare by the Director, Office of Emergency Planning.

(4) In the event of a national emergency, the total reserves of blood products, artificial plasma volume expanders and related items shall be subject to immediate reallocation by Executive order.

(d) *Emergency allocation of blood and blood derivatives.* The Director, Office of Emergency Planning, may, in an emergency, allocate blood collected by organizations actively participating in this Program. With modifications dependent on the magnitude and type of emergency, the following priorities will be applied:

(1) First priority shall be given to the allocation of blood to the Armed Services for whole blood transfusion purposes.

(2) Second priority shall be given to the allocation of whole blood and blood derivatives for civilian needs.

(e) *Recruitment of volunteer blood donors.* When directed by the Office of Emergency Planning, the total donor recruitment program shall be geared to soliciting donors for the Blood Program as a whole rather than for specific parts of the whole. The various agencies involved in this program shall unite in a coordinated effort to inform the people clearly of the urgent need for blood. The Office of Emergency Planning shall designate the agency to administer this effort.

6. *Responsibilities.* (a) The Office of Emergency Planning will exercise authoritative coordination of the program. It will develop and promulgate overall policy guidance and will adjudicate conflicts between participating Federal agencies. The Health Resources Advisory Committee, with the assistance of the Committee on Blood, will assist the Director, Office of Emergency Planning, in the discharge of these responsibilities.

(b) The Department of Defense is responsible for administering the military aspects of this program.

(c) The Department of Health, Education, and Welfare is responsible for the nonmilitary aspects of as part of its assignment of responsibility for planning the mobilization of the nation's civilian health resources.

(d) The Secretary of Defense maintain an interagency coordinate Federal agency programing aspects for research development projects relating to national Emergency Blood Program to best support that program. This mission should not be controlled or direction of the research agency represented on this.

(e) The National Research shall:

(1) Formulate, evaluate and recommend programs and projects primarily to scientific aspects of national Emergency Blood Program.

(2) Recommend actions to be taken by the various agencies in the operation of the National Emergency Blood Program based on research determinations.

7. *Interagency research.* (a) Funds shall be provided the operation of the National Research Council in connection with the National Emergency Blood Program by participating agencies in accordance with established procedures.

(b) Interested Federal agencies, as the Office of Emergency Planning, Department of Defense, Public Health Service, and the Food and Drug Administration, shall seek the advice of the Research Council on problems primarily to the scientific research and Development Program for Emergency Blood Program.

(c) The National Research Council, the Department of Defense Committee, and the Office of Emergency Planning shall keep each other informed of program developments.

8. *Reporting.* (a) Reports of activities of the Council and Committee shall be submitted when requested by the Office of Emergency Planning.

(b) As and when directed by the Office of Emergency Planning, the Department of Health, Education, and the Department of Defense, the Office of Emergency Planning reports covering (1) the requirements and reserves of program items; and (2) related.

Dated: April 10, 1967.

FARRIS
Director
Emergency

[F.R. Doc. 67-4145; Filed, 8:46 a.m.]

Attachment 1-4.

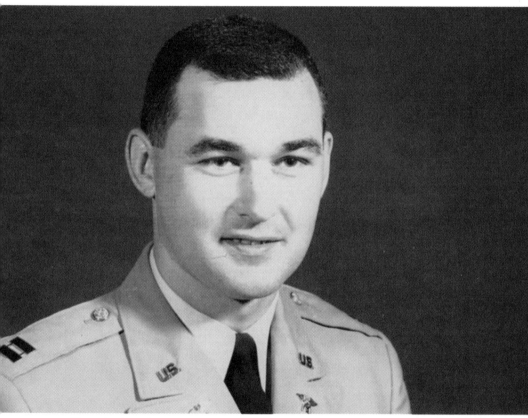
Figure 2-1. Captain James Spiker Jr. 1966. Courtesy of Colonel (Ret) James Spiker Jr.

CHAPTER TWO

Blood Program Growth, Standardization, and Coordination: 1960s

Although it was shaped in large part by the Vietnam War, the Army Blood Program also built on significant developments during the 1960s before the war. Three crucial pillars of success included program growth, standardized processes, and operational coordination. Advances and standardization in blood screening, increased capacity for collection and shipment, uniform blood handling processes, and education about the importance of blood donation all contributed to the growth of the program. An emphasis on operational coordination ensured that the numerous advances in technology and program management were shared among all Army Blood Program stakeholders.

EARLY 1960s

With a goal of standardizing operations, the Department of Defense (DoD) released operational procedures for military blood donor centers. The focus was on the collection of whole blood, processing, and shipment. With consistent processes, military leaders thought that blood could be exchanged among the hospitals of all three services without concern. The manual also included standardized equipment, supplies, and forms.[1] Staff from donor centers and blood banks used a standard form, DD Form 572, *Blood Donor Record Card*, to screen potential donors. The 1960 edition of DD Form 572 (Exhibit 2-1) added a section for tracking the disposition of the blood to the 1955 edition. Standardization proved to be the correct approach when the FDA later began regulating the US blood industry facilities as biological and pharmaceutical facilities.

26 A HISTORY OF THE ARMY BLOOD PROGRAM

Exhibit 2-1: Department of Defense. *Blood Donor Record Card*. Washington, DC: DOD; 1960. Department of Defense Form 572.

Dr. J. Portnoy developed the rapid plasma reagin (RPR) test, a nontreponemal assay for syphilis (known to be transmitted through blood transfusions), in 1961. This new assay eventually replaced the earlier serologic tests for syphilis. One of the earlier tests was the Kahn test, dating to 1922. It used macroscopic flocculation without complement, but unfortunately the Kahn test did not have a standardized antigen. Researchers standardized the antigen in 1946, which led to the development of cardiolipin microflocculation tests, such as the venereal disease research laboratory (VDRL) test.[2]

Figure 2-1 shows Captain James Spiker Jr. (later a member of the US Army Blood Bank Fellowship [BBF] class of '65–66), who arrived at the 121st Evacuation Hospital in Korea as a clinical laboratory officer in March 1962. At this time, the blood bank section was collecting and processing blood at the hospital. Mobile blood drives were conducted at local Army Support Command units near Inchon and during weekly trips to either Seoul Military Hospital or forward camps in I Corps. Staff transportation to most mobile blood drives in I Corps was by helicopter. The collection site furnished donor beds and postdonation refreshments. The donor collection team often carried whiskey obtained from the hospital pharmacy, authorized for use to those who wanted a "shot" after donating. The 121st shipped processed blood to Seoul Military Hospital and the two combat support hospitals in I Corps, as well as to Korean hospitals and (less often) to the 11th Evacuation Hospital in Pusan. No blood was shipped in from outside Korea. The clinical laboratory officer at the 121st was the 8th Army Blood Program officer (as an additional duty), who coordinated blood collections with the 8th Army chief of operations. A regulation on blood programs provided authorization and limited guidance, according to Colonel (Retired) Jim Spiker in his email communication dated June 2014.

On May 15, 1962, the DoD issued DoD Directive 6480.5, *Department of Defense Blood Program* (Attachment 2-1).[3] This document directed the secretary of the Army to establish an organization with the responsibilities of coordinating blood activities of the military departments under the DoD Blood Program. The Military Blood Program Agency (MBPA) was established as a part of the Office of The Surgeon General by General Order Number 28, established July 17, 1962.[4] The MBPA was to "accomplish under the direction and control of the Secretary of Defense the joint aspects of the Department of Defense Blood Program as defined in DoD Directive 6480.5."[4] Within the Office of The Surgeon General, the MBPA operated under the staff supervision of the director of plans, supply, and operations, and was physically located in the Main Navy

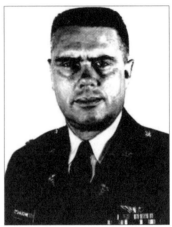

Figure 2-2. Lieutenant Colonel Edward O'Shaughnessy, first director of the Military Blood Program Agency. Courtesy of the Armed Services Blood Program Office.

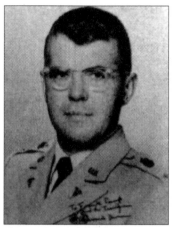

Figure 2-3. Colonel William Crosby, Medical Corps. 1973. Reproduced from: Camp FR, Conte N, Brewer JR. *Military Blood Banking 1941-1973 — Lessons Learned Applicable to Civil Disasters and Other Considerations.* Ft Knox, Kentucky: US Army Medical Research Laboratory; 1973.

Building, Room 2827, in Washington, DC. Lieutenant Colonel Edward O'Shaughnessy, Medical Corps, US Army (Figure 2-2), was the first director, serving from 1962 through 1964. General Order Number 36, released on August 23, 1962, placed the Army element of the MBPA under the US Army Medical Service Field Activities unit, Walter Reed Army Medical Center, with logistical support to be provided by the Office of The Surgeon General, according to Colonel (Retired) Tony Polk's email communication dated March 2014. During its initial year, the MBPA developed a mobilization plan to provide whole blood during emergencies. The first implementation of this plan occurred during the Cuban missile crisis in October 1962.[4]

Incident to the establishment of the MBPA and reassignment of functions formerly assigned to the Armed Services Medical Material Coordinating Committee, a question arose in the late summer and fall of 1962 regarding the dividing line of authority and responsibility between the Defense Medical Material Board (which replaced the Armed Services Medical Material Coordinating Committee) and the MBPA. The questions related particularly to policy and action regarding acceptability, distribution, and use of blood and substitutes, disposition of stockpile items, and classification and review of standard stock items related to the blood programs. By mid-September 1962 an impasse was reached between the MBPA director and the Defense Medical Material Board chairman. On September 19, 1962, Lieutenant Colonel Edward O'Shaughnessy wrote a memorandum to the deputy assistant secretary of defense (health and medical) requesting clarification of the roles of the two agencies. Two weeks later on October 1, the Honorable Frank B. Berry replied to both agencies, resolving the main areas of policy, according to Colonel (Retired) Tony Polk's email communication dated March 2014. The next edition of DoD Directive 6480.5, released in 1972, specified that the Military Blood Program Office (previously known as the MBPA) would coordinate with the Defense Medical Material Board on essential characteristics of material associated with military blood banking.[5]

The Army included a blood program section in Army Regulation (AR) 40-3, *Medical Service—Medical, Dental, and Veterinary Care*, released in 1962.[6]

The regulation addressed the Army Blood Program, which included the command (local) blood program, the distribution of whole blood and its fractions to Army hospitals, and a research and development program to advance and improve the entire program. One paragraph discusses blood for transfusion purposes and states that the "payment of donors is authorized at the prevailing rate," not to exceed $50 for a single donation.[6] The practice of using paid donors eventually ended in 1973.

The Army Medical Service Mobilization Plan, dated November 11, 1963, established the requirement for a blood transfusion service.[7] The following year, Colonel William Crosby, Medical Corps (Figure 2-3), and Major Frank Camp, Medical Service Corps (BBF class of '60–61) (Figure 2-4), were both assigned to the Walter Reed Army Institute of Research in Washington, DC. They conducted a staff study to determine whether there was a requirement to establish a blood transfusion service center for the US Army. They believed that readiness would be greatly improved with a center adequately staffed, located in a troop concentration area, and with adequate communication to permit economical shipment of blood. The study proposed a US Army blood transfusion service center that would have a donor center, a blood group reference laboratory, a training center, and a research laboratory. Three sites were recommended: (1) Ft Knox, (2) Ft Sam Houston, and (3) the Presidio of San Francisco. Ft Knox was subsequently selected, and the program was established there under the Army Medical Research Laboratory.[7] Beginning on July 1, 1965, Major Camp served as the first director of this program, remaining for 10 years.[8]

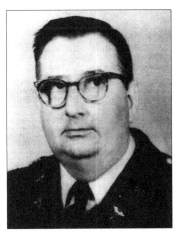

Figure 2-4. Lieutenant Colonel Frank Camp Jr. Photograph from Camp Memorial Blood Center closure files.

In 1964 Brigadier General Kendrick published a book called *Blood Program in World War II*.[9] This book has become a valuable resource for the modern Army Blood Program because it outlines the history of blood banking before World War II, and it highlights critical challenges and key advancements of military blood bank during and after the war.

The Army released specific guidance, AR 600-12, *Blood Donor Procurement Program*, for procuring blood donors in the Washington metropolitan area early in 1965.[10] AR 600-12 established responsibilities, policies, and procedures for donor recruitment at Army installations in the area in support of the American National Red Cross as part of the DoD Blood Program. Walter Reed Army Medical Center and the Dewitt Army Hospital operated their own procurement programs. The DoD Washington-area blood donor coordinator provided guidance to the Army hospital programs. The division of the Washington metropolitan area, later known as the Military District of Washington, continued into the 1980s.

VIETNAM WAR

During the post–Korean War period of the 1950s and 1960s, the United States was concerned about the spread of communism. Ho Chi Minh, the communist leader of North Vietnam, wanted to unite all of Vietnam under one rule. Under President Dwight Eisenhower and President John Kennedy, the United States provided advisors to South Vietnam. Lyndon Johnson assumed the presidency after Kennedy's death in November 1963. On August 2, 1964, North Vietnamese vessels attacked American ships in the Gulf of Tonkin. Just 5 days later, on August 7, Congress passed the Gulf of Tonkin Resolution authorizing the president to use any means necessary to protect US interests in the region. By the end of 1965, the US had nearly 200,000 troops in South Vietnam. By 1969, there were 480,000 troops.[11]

The large number of troops fighting in Vietnam and the urgent blood product requirements tested the military blood program's ability to support a major operation. Thus, the Vietnam War played a huge role in the development of a coordinated collection, transportation, and distribution system for this and future wars.

The 406th Medical Laboratory commander served as the Pacific Theater blood program officer.[12] According to the 406th Mobile Medical Laboratory 1965 semi-annual report, the blood bank collected blood from American donors in Japan, Korea, and Okinawa.[13] The blood was processed at the 406th Medical Laboratory in Japan for shipment to the central blood bank in Saigon. Sub-depots were established in Nha Trang, Qui Nhon, and Da Nang for further distribution.

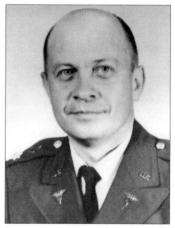

Figure 2-5. In 1965, Major William Collins designed a new blood shipping box made of Styrofoam because the current fiberboard shipping box did not perform well in the heat and humidity of Vietnam. Courtesy of Mr. Bill Turcan, US Army Blood Bank Fellowship.

Only low-titer type O whole blood was used because it was ideal for emergency situations or when a service member's blood type was unknown. But as the war escalated, type-specific blood was incorporated into the theater inventories.

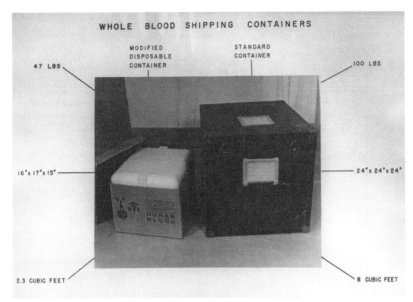

Figure 2-6. Comparison of Collins new blood shipping box and the current blood shipping box. Courtesy of Major (Ret) H. Curt Harrell.

In 1965, Major William S. Collins II (Figure 2-5) (BBF class of '58–59), director of the 406th Medical Laboratory and Blood Bank in Japan, introduced a modified disposable blood shipping box made of Styrofoam for the shipping and distribution of blood. The previously used fiberboard box did not perform well in extreme heat and humidity. The new container, which became known as the Collins box, was smaller than the standard shipping container—2.3 ft^3 (16 in. × 17 in. × 15 in.) compared to 8 ft^3 (24 in. × 24 in. × 24 in.) (Figure 2-6). The new box had a Styrofoam insert with nine compartments (Figure 2-7). The Styrofoam container, with 38-mm sides, could maintain appropriate shipping temperatures for up to 48 hours—twice as long as the previous storage box—and it cost less money ($1.40 compared to $100) and weighed less (Figures 2-8 to 2-13). It provided flexibility for blood bankers around the world because it did not need to be returned.[14] Collins worked with local businesses in Japan to produce the new container. Through the end of 1968, Japan was the only procurement source of these shipping boxes for the DoD. It was not until 1969 that the DoD awarded a contract to American companies. The first American order was for 12,000 shipping boxes.[12]

In the summer of 1966 the requirement for blood quickly began to exceed the capacity of the 406th. During this time of increasing requirements, the US Pacific Command sent a request to the MBPA to assist with the shortfalls in

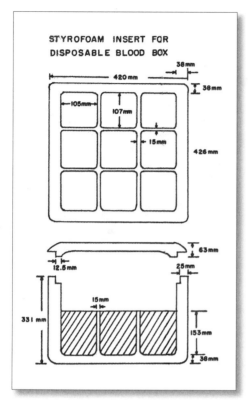

Figure 2-7. Collins Box Styrofoam Design and Study. Courtesy of Major (Ret) H. Curt Harrell.

theater (the requirement went from 100 units per month in early 1965 to over 38,000 units per month in 1969). To help meet the increasing demand for blood in Vietnam, the MBPA assigned quotas to the three services. The agency also established a new tri-service unit, called the Armed Services Whole Blood Processing Laboratory (ASWBPL), at McGuire Air Force Base (AFB) in New Jersey to process units of blood collected in the United States and prepare them for shipment overseas (Figures 2-14 to 2-16). Processing meant not only verifying the blood group and Rh type, but also determining the titer of the type O whole blood. From the ASWBPL, the blood was shipped through the blood transshipment center at Elmendorf AFB to the Yokota transshipment center in Japan. The main 406th Medical Laboratory went to Yokota and brought the blood to Camp Zama, performed a third blood group and type on all group O blood, and then re-iced the blood and took it back to Yokota AFB. From Japan the blood was flown to the US Army Vietnam Central Blood Bank.[14]

Before whole blood could be flown to the ASWBPL for processing and shipment into Vietnam, the Army had to coordinate with its 17 active blood donor centers in continental United States.[8] These sites were as follows:

- Ft Benning, Georgia
- Ft Bliss, Texas
- Ft Bragg, North Carolina
- Ft Campbell, Kentucky
- Ft Devens, Massachusetts
- Ft Dix, New Jersey
- Ft Gordon, Georgia

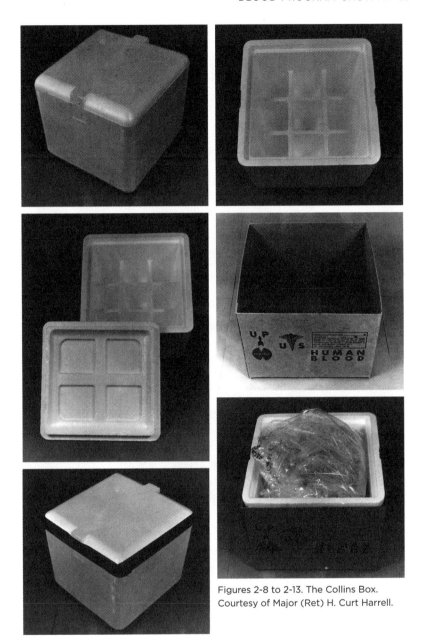

Figures 2-8 to 2-13. The Collins Box.
Courtesy of Major (Ret) H. Curt Harrell.

- Ft Hood, Texas
- Ft Jackson, South Carolina
- Ft Knox, Kentucky
- Ft Lee, Virginia
- Ft Leonard Wood, Missouri
- Ft Lewis, Washington
- Ft Ord, California
- Ft Polk, Louisiana
- Ft Sam Houston, Texas
- Ft Sill, Oklahoma

The Army established the donor center at Ft Dix, New Jersey, to make up for shortfalls in meeting the theater requirements. Two key reasons for selecting this post were that it was a large basic training installation and it was close to McGuire AFB. Collected blood was processed at the Walson Army Hospital and then delivered to the ASWBPL.[15] Blood was provided to hospitals in the continental United States from three Army donor centers: (1) the Blood Transfusion Division of the US Army Medical Research Laboratory, Ft Knox, provided blood to the Walter Reed General Hospital; (2) the donor center at Ft Dix supported Valley Forge General Hospital at Phoenixville, Pennsylvania, and Dunham Army Hospital at Carlisle Barracks, Pennsylvania; and (3) Ft Leonard Wood, Missouri's donor center sent blood to Fitzsimons Army Hospital in Aurora, Colorado.[12]

During the summer of 1966, Lieutenant Colonel Camp led a group O blood verification mission to Ft Benning, Georgia. The mission was to take a team and equipment to verify blood groups of the 1st Cavalry Division (Airmobile), which was preparing to deploy to the Central Highlands area of South Vietnam. The division was expected to be on the tail of a very long medical supply chain. Lieutenant Colonel Camp, the three current blood bank fellows (Captain Jerry Brewer, Captain Jack Rodgers, and Captain James Spiker) and a noncommissioned officer, Sergeant Louis Agiliu, comprised the team, and their equipment consisted of test tubes, racks, applicator sticks, and highly potent anti-sera. No centrifugation was done. Specimens coagulated while sitting at room temperature. Approximately 3,200 soldiers were verified as group O. Their dog tags were stamped "UD" for universal donor, according to Colonel (Retired) Jim Spiker's email dated June 2014.

A blood donor center with the capability of collecting, processing, and shipping 500 units per month of whole blood was established at Brooke Army Medical Center in December 1966. Major Matthew Gottlieb (BBF class of '61–62) was tasked to provide blood to the newly established ASWBPL at McGuire AFB to help meet the blood requirements in Vietnam. After finding an empty, wooden, two-story barracks near the current Army Medical Department

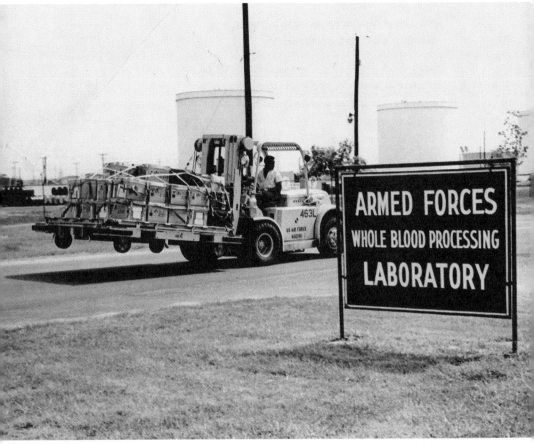

Figure 2-14. The Armed Services Whole Blood Processing Laboratory (ASWBPL) at McGuire Air Force Base, 1967. Courtesy of Colonel (Ret) Anthony Polk.

Center and School (AMEDDC&S) on Ft Sam Houston, Gottlieb and Captain Anthony Polk (later, BBF class of '72–73) wrote the first Brooke Army Medical Center Blood Donor Center regulations. This required the installation engineers to refurbish the empty barracks for the Medical Field Service School (which had moved from Carlisle Barracks to Ft Sam Houston in 1946), to provide a facility that could accommodate donors on a continuous basis. The barracks, Building T-1126 on Lawton Road, was converted into a blood donor facility at a cost of $24,987. This was the genesis of organized blood collections on Ft Sam Houston.[16]

Back in theater, the 9th Medical Lab, located on the Tan Son Nhut Air Base outside Saigon, served as a reference and central laboratory for Army hospitals in Vietnam. The US Army Republic of Vietnam Central Blood Bank was originally

```
ARMED SERVICES WHOLE BLOOD PROCESSING LABORATORY

PERSONNEL ROSTER ON 18 SEPTEMBER 1967

FIRST ROW:                          (ALL LISTINGS ARE FROM LEFT TO RIGHT)

ENS DONALD R. LEVAN, MSC, USNR - LABORATORY OFFICER
CAPT ROBERT J. SARNOWSKI, USAF, MC - OFFICER IN CHARGE
HMC ARVID E. HEIMANN, USN - NON-COMMISSIONED OFFICER IN CHARGE   8417-LABORATORY

SECOND ROW:

TSGT GERALD A. BROWN, USAF         90470-LABORATORY
HM2 JOHN A. STERN, USN             8417-LABORATORY
A2C LEONARD J. SWEDER, USAF        90450-LABORATORY
A3C RICHARD J. CARTER, USAF RES    90630-ADMINISTRATIVE (DUTY IN LABORATORY)
SP-4 ROBERT E. DEVINE, USA         92B20-LABORATORY

THIRD ROW:

SSGT ALBERT L. FABOZZI, USAF       90450-LABORATORY
SP-4 RALPH N. FRASER, USA          92B20-LABORATORY
A3C ANTHONY LONGO, USAF RES        90530-PHARMACY (DUTY IN LABORATORY)
SP-4 RONALD X. BERNARDI, USA       92B20-LABORATORY
SSGT ANTHONY J. BEASLY, USAF       90470-LABORATORY (TDY)

FOURTH ROW:

HM2 RONALD E. ROBERTS, USN         8417-LABORATORY
A1C ALLEN L. BELL, USAF            90650-ADMINISTRATIVE
SP-4 JOSEPH W. TAYLOR, JR., USA    76K20-MACHINE GUNNER (DUTY IN LABORATORY)
YN3 EDWARD T. MILLER, USN          2500-ADMINISTRATIVE
A3C LARRY B. SPERO, USAF RES       91530-SUPPLY

MISSING FROM PHOTOGRAPH:

SP-4 MARK T. KURDONIK, USA         92B20-LABORATORY - ON LEAVE
PFC GEORGE J. CLARK, USA           76K10-MACHINE GUNNER (DUTY IN LABORATORY)
                                   - ON NIGHT DUTY
```

Figure 2-15A. The staff of the Armed Services Whole Blood Processing Laboratory, 1967. Courtesy of Colonel (Ret) Anthony Polk.

attached to the 9th Medical Lab. It managed the distribution of blood to US military hospitals and subdepots throughout Vietnam. However, in 1969 it was moved to an island on Cam Ranh Bay with the 6th Convalescent Center. This was mainly because, after the 1968 Tet Offensive, there was a concern about the enemy gaining the area around Saigon and Tan Son Nhut and disrupting the critical blood supply route, according to Colonel (Retired) Anthony Polk's email, dated August 2011.

The 406th Medical Company (Blood Bank) was authorized three numbered blood detachments, each with a blood bank officer (Figure 2-17) and three laboratory officers. However, the 406th leadership viewed its entire organization as one big team (Figures 2-18 and 2-19). Most of the personnel assigned to the detachments worked in other laboratory departments until they conducted a blood drive. The team traveled to every installation in Japan and made periodic trips to Okinawa, Korea, the Philippines, and Guam. The blood collected in the

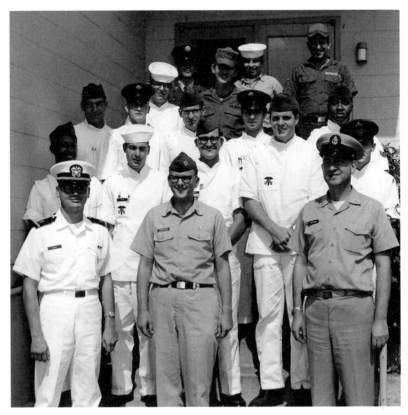

Figure 2-15B. The staff of the Armed Services Whole Blood Processing Laboratory, 1967. Courtesy of Colonel (Ret) Anthony Polk.

Pacific Command area of responsibility mostly went to the hospitals in the Pacific Command communications zone (Figure 2-20). In Japan there were four 1,000-bed Army hospitals in the Tokyo area, two 500-bed Air Force hospitals, and two 500-bed Navy hospitals. The 406th also shipped blood to the 121st Evacuation Hospital in Korea, the Army hospital on Okinawa, Clark AFB in the Philippines, and Air Force and Navy hospitals on Guam. Additionally, it supplemented continental US blood shipments to Vietnam as required. When Captain Loran McKinley (later, BBF class of '71–72) arrived on Okinawa, he began his own blood collections, and Captain John Bell (later, BBF class of '73–74) in Korea did the same. However, McKinley and Bell sent testing to the 406th because it was a centralized testing facility in 1970, according to Colonel (Retired) Anthony Polk's email dated August 2011.

During the war, the Army did not use any frozen red blood cells because of the need for large, heavy equipment; sufficient staff with the specific training to

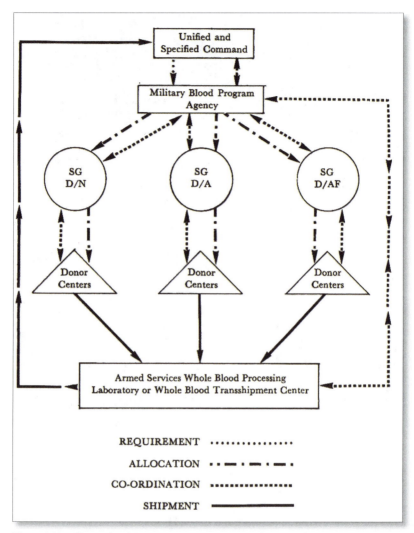

Figure 2-16. Military Blood Program Agency operational scheme for whole blood shipped through the Armed Services Whole Blood Processing Laboratory (ASWBPL) at McGuire AFB, 1966–1970. The wire diagram shows how the newly formed ASWBPL fits into the blood distribution system. Blood is collected by military blood donor centers and shipped to the ASWBPL. There, the blood types of the units would be verified, and antibodies titered. On completion of these steps, the blood would be repackaged for shipment to the Unified or Combatant Command. Reproduced from: Neel S. *Medical Support of the US Army in Vietnam 1965-1970*. Washington, DC: Department of the Army; 1991.

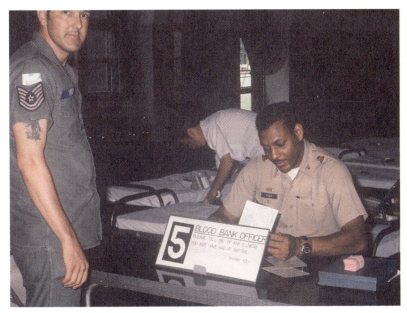

Figure 2-17. Captain Anthony Polk, US Forces Japan blood collecting team, 1971. Courtesy of Colonel (Ret) Anthony Polk.

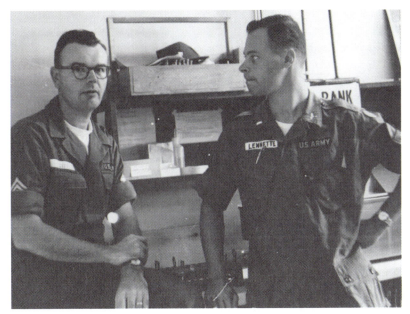

Figure 2-18. 406th Mobile Medical Laboratory (Blood Bank) at Nha Trang, Vietnam. Sergeant First Class Francis Guy and First Lieutenant Paul Lennette discussing blood needs for mass casualties in December 1965. Courtesy of Major (Ret) H. Curt Harrell.

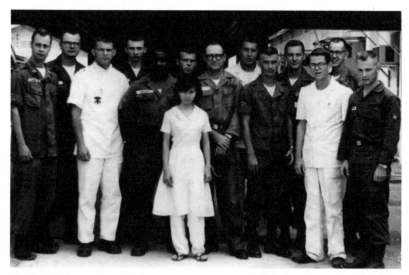

Figure 2-19. Some the staff of the 406th Mobile Medical Laboratory in Vietnam—First Lieutenant Lennette, Sergeant First Class Guy, Private First Class Cooley, Specialist 4th Class Ferguson, Specialist 5th Class Matthews, Miss Ha, SP4 Rolland, SP5 Taylor, Specialist 4th Class Jablonski, SP5 Williams, Specialist 4th Class Albert, Private First Class Machen, Major Frank Kiel (Commander), and Specialist 4th Class Thompson. Courtesy of Major (Ret) H. Curt Harrell.

deglycerolize the frozen units; and a stable environment. Instead, the belief was that research and funding should be directed toward extending the shelf life of red blood cells. The Navy, however, saw potential utility in using deglycerolized red blood cells in treating combat-wounded casualities.[17] During a brief period in 1966, the Navy transfused more than 450 units of deglycerolized red blood cells at the Naval Station Hospital Da Nang. This was the first use of frozen red blood cells on the battlefield.[18]

At the height of American involvement in the Vietnam War, blood used to support the effort was collected at military installations in the Pacific and the United States. On average, it took 7 days for blood collected at continental US military donor centers to reach the theater of operations. As US involvement peaked, blood use steadily increased, as did use of the new modified shipping container and coordination between blood centers and the theater. The Vietnam War was also the first time that the ARC was not needed to supplement blood support to the operational theater. Instead, the military blood donor centers collected the blood free of charge from military personnel, civilians at military locations, and service members' families who generously wanted to support the military.[14] Attachment 2-2 shows examples of publicity and marketing efforts used

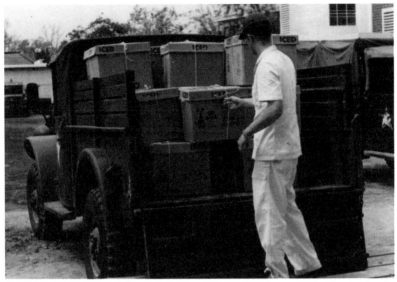

Figure 2-20. 406th Blood Bank in Vietnam—Private First Class Troha loading 500 units of blood for Marias in Donong. Courtesy of Major (Ret) H. Curt Harrell.

to encourage voluntary, unpaid blood donation. At the conclusion of the war, nearly 2 million units were collected by military blood donor centers in the United States and the Pacific Theater. The blood usage was 4.0 to 5.0 units per casualty, with an average of 4.4 units per casualty.[8] The Army eventually deactivated the 406th Medical Company (Blood Bank) in 1976 according to Colonel (Retired) Jim Spiker's email dated June 2014.

SUMMARY

Improvements in shipping and distribution, along with the establishment of the MBPA to coordinate the efforts of the Services' Blood Program proved that the military could be self-sustaining in support military operations overseas. This crucial capability directly affected battlefield wound survivorship rates.

REFERENCES

1. US Departments of the Army, Navy, and Air Force. *Operational Procedures for the Military Blood Donor Centers*. Washington, DC: Department of Defense; 1959. Technical Manual 8-255, NAVMED P-5064, AFM 160-16.
2. Centers for Disease Control and Prevention. History of diagnostic tests for syphilis. http://www.cdc.gov/std/syphilis/manual-1998/CHAPT1A2.pdf. Accessed June 1, 2016.

3. US Department of Defense. *Department of Defense Blood Program*. Washington, DC: DoD; 1962. DoD Directive 6480.5.
4. US Department of the Army. *Annual Report of the Surgeon General, United States Army 1958/59–1962/63*. Washington, DC: DA, Office of The Surgeon General; 1963. http://babel.hathitrust.org/cgi/pt?q1=Military%20blood%20program%20agency;id=uc1.b3098772;view=1up;seq=772;start=1;sz=10;page=search;num=36#view=1up;seq=772. Updated February 17, 2012. Accessed June 1, 2016.
5. US Department of Defense. *Military Blood Program*. Washington, DC: DoD; 1972. DoD Directive 6480.5.
6. US Department of the Army. *Medical Service – Medical, Dental, and Veterinary Care*. Washington, DC: DA; 1962. Army Regulation 40-3.
7. US Department of the Army. *US Army Blood Transfusion Service Center*. Washington, DC: DA, Walter Reed Army Institute of Research; 1964. Staff study.
8. Camp FR, Conte N, Brewer JR. *Military Blood Banking 1941–1973–Lessons Learned Applicable to Civil Disasters and Other Considerations*. Fort Knox, KY: US Army Medical Research Laboratory, Blood Bank Center; 1973.
9. Kendrick DB. *Blood Program in World War II*. Washington, DC: Department of the Army; 1964.
10. US Department of the Army. *Blood Donor Procurement Program*. Washington, DC: DA; 1962. Army Regulation 600-12.
11. Trueman CN. Timeline of the Vietnam War. The History Learning Site. The Vietnam War website. http://www.historylearningsite.co.uk/vietnam-war/timeline-of-the-vietnam-war/. Accessed June 1, 2016.
12. US Department of the Army. *Annual Report of the Surgeon General, United States Army 1965/66–1967/68*. Washington, DC: DA, Office of The Surgeon General; 1968. http://babel.hathitrust.org/cgi/pt?q1=shipping;id=uc1.b3108013;view=1up;seq=56;num=40;start=1;sz=10;page=search#view=1up;seq=56. Published March 23, 2014. Accessed June 1, 2016.
13. 406th Mobile Medical Laboratory. *Semi-Annual Report*. APO San Francisco: 406th Mobile Medical Laboratory; July 1, 1965 – December 31, 1965. Located at: Archives room, US Army Medical Department Museum, Ft Sam Houston, TX.
14. Neel SH. *Medical Support of the US Army in Vietnam 1965–1970*. Washington, DC: Department of the Army; 1991.
15. Pellegrini J. Vietnam War era blood operations help shape modern day ASBP. United States Military Blood Program website. http://www.militaryblood.dod.mil/viewcontent.aspx?con_id_pk=1587. Published April 7, 2014. Accessed June 1, 2016.
16. Brooke Army Medical Center. *Army Medical Service Activities Report*. Fort Sam Houston, TX; 1966. http://stimson.contentdm.oclc.org/cdm/singleitem/collection/p16379coll5/id/10/rec/12. Accessed June 1, 2016.
17. Crosby WH. Frozen blood for a military transfusion service. *Mil Med*. 1967;132(2):119–121.
18. Spinella PC, Dunne J, Beilman GJ, et al. Constant challenges and evolution of US military transfusion medicine and blood operations in combat. *Transfusion*. 2012;52:1146–1153.

May 15, 1962
NUMBER **6480.5**

ASD(M)

Department of Defense Directive

SUBJECT Department of Defense Blood Program

References: (a) DoD Directive 6480.1, "National Blood Program," August 20, 1953 (hereby cancelled)
(b) "National Blood Program, Statement of Basic Principles," issued by the Office of Civil and Defense Mobilization (now, Office of Emergency Planning), November 9, 1960

I. PURPOSE

This Directive (1) defines the Department of Defense Blood Program and assigns responsibilities for carrying out its provisions; (2) assigns to the Secretary of the Army certain responsibilities for joint aspects of the Department of Defense Blood Program, to be executed on a joint staff basis, under the direction and control of the Secretary of Defense.

II. APPLICABILITY AND SCOPE

The provisions of this Directive apply to the military departments and the unified and specified commands, and cover the collection, processing and distribution of whole blood and its fractions, under all degrees of emergency conditions.

III. CANCELLATION

Reference (a) is hereby superseded and cancelled.

IV. DEFINITIONS

As used in this Directive, Department of Defense Blood Program means the blood programs of the military departments and of the

Attachment 2-1.

unified and specified commands, and the structure necessary to integrate these programs in time of national emergency. It includes the following functions:

1. The collection at military installations, the processing, and the distribution of whole blood and its fractions to military hospitals on a local or regional basis.

2. The procurement of whole blood, for military use, from sources outside the Department of Defense.

3. The maintenance and implementation of plans to provide for the collection, processing, and distribution of whole blood and its fractions to the Armed Forces, world-wide, under all degrees of emergency conditions.

4. The provision and maintenance of a source of trained personnel, facilities, and supplies and equipment, adequate to meet initial emergency requirements.

5. A research and development program devoted to progress and improvement in the areas of blood, blood derivatives, and plasma volume expanders, and the techniques, facilities and materiel related thereto.

V. RESPONSIBILITIES

A. The Secretary of the Army is responsible for:

1. Assigning to a specific, identifiable organizational activity within his department the responsibilities and functions listed in subparagraphs a. through j., below.

2. Providing for joint staffing of the designated activity by medical service representatives of the Army, Navy, and Air Force who shall be selected by and have direct access to their respective Surgeons General.

3. Providing adequate administrative support for the designated activity.

The following responsibilities and functions are to be executed by the designated activity:

a. Implementing the DoD Blood Program policy guidance established by the Assistant Secretary of Defense (Manpower).

Attachment 2-1. Continued

May 15, 62
6480.5

b. Maintaining and disseminating plans for coordinating the collection, processing and distribution of blood and blood products necessary to meet requirements beyond the capability of the military department or command concerned, and directing the implementation of such plans.

c. Coordinating and integrating the plans, policies, and procedures of the military departments, and unified and specified commands under the DoD Blood Program, to the extent necessary to assure the effectiveness of the plans referred to in b., above.

d. Coordinating DoD Blood Program plans and actions which have military operational implications with the Joint Chiefs of Staff.

e. Providing the Defense Supply Agency with technical and professional operational guidance on the procurement of whole blood and fractions, when required, and on mobilization and industrial mobilization requirements for plasma expanders, both natural and synthetic.

f. Providing direct DoD liaison with other Government agencies having an interest in blood and related items.

g. Developing and promulgating policies (fully coordinated with the military departments) on:

   (1) The collection, procurement, processing, storage, distribution, and use of whole blood.

   (2) The acceptability, distribution, and use of blood fractions and synthetic or other non-human plasma volume expanders.

h. Obtaining and maintaining, on a continuing basis, emergency and mobilization military requirements of whole blood from the military departments and commands, as appropriate; and determining net DoD requirements.

i. Receiving all requisitions for emergency quantities of whole blood from overseas, and from Continental United States, when quantities required exceed local resources.

j. Establishing on behalf of the Director of Defense Research and Engineering a central register of military

Attachment 2-1. Continued

department research and development projects on blood, blood derivatives, and plasma volume expanders to prevent unnecessary duplication and overlapping of effort.

B. The Secretaries of the Army, Navy, and Air Force, and the Commanders of unified and specified commands, are responsible for:

1. Maintaining internal departmental and command Blood Programs. These Programs shall provide for the collection, or other means of procurement, of whole blood and its fractions at military installations; and for processing and distributing these products to meet (a) normal departmental or command requirements, and (b) within their capabilities, requirements generated by military operations as well as local, regional, or national emergencies.

2. Insuring that their respective Blood Programs reflect the policies established herein, and the guidance to be developed by the designated activity referred to in V.A.1.

3. Insuring that the organizational structure of their blood programs can be readily expanded and integrated with the joint program when necessary.

4. Submitting requirements and reporting capabilities, as requested, to the designated activity referred to in V.A.1.

C. The Assistant Secretary of Defense (Manpower) is responsible for providing overall policy guidance on the DoD Blood Program, and for coordinating it with the National Blood Program, when required.

D. The Director, Defense Research and Engineering is responsible for coordinating and issuing policy guidance on military department research and development projects related to the DoD Blood Program.

VI. GENERAL

In carrying out the responsibilities set forth above, the Secretary of the Army is authorized to communicate directly with commanders of unified and specified commands, subject to the requirements of V.A. .d., above.

Attachment 2-1. Continued

May 15, 62
6480.5

VII. **EFFECTIVE DATE AND IMPLEMENTATION**

This Directive is effective June 1, 1962. Within thirty (30) days of receipt of this Directive (1) The Secretaries of the Army, Navy and Air Force shall develop such implementing instructions as are appropriate to their departments and (2) the Secretary of the Army shall develop, in collaboration with the Secretaries of the Navy and Air Force, implementing instructions for the joint aspects of the Directive. All implementing instructions will be submitted to the Assistant Secretary of Defense (Manpower) for approval. After approval and publication, two copies of the implementing regulations shall be submitted to the Assistant Secretary of Defense (Manpower).

Roswell Gilpatric
Deputy Secretary of Defense

MILITARY BLOOD PROGRAM

1. Listed below are excerpts from daily bulletins, newspaper editorials, posters, etc, which might give you some ideas for use with publicity concerning the Whole Blood Program:

   a. Today, just as yesterday, our American brothers are dying on the battle fields of the Republic of Vietnam. We are appealing to your patriotic sense of duty to help them in thier great struggle. ... Our community now is not only faced with the task of supplying materials but blood as well. We are now, as we always have been, in need of blood.... We simply ask you not to let our men down... We are located... Our hours of operation are.... We appreciate your past support and know you will continue to aid us in the future.

   b. Blood is like ammunition, it needs to be available before the action begins or before the casulties come in order to save lives. Unlike ammunition, it cannot be saved indefinitely. Donate now.

   c. You wouldn't refuse to receive a pint of blood, why refuse to donate one.

   d. Join the Life Saver Club, donate a pint of blood.

   e. "Ask not what you can do for your country" -- do it -- by giving a pint of blood.

   f. Your blood donation is urgently needed now.

   g. Give a gift of life during the holiday season.

   h. The blood you give helps someone to live.

   i. You can give the ultimate gift this Christmas season. Give the gift of life, a pint of blood, now.

   j. Blood is like ammunition, it needs to be available at the aid station before the action begins or before the casulties come in, in order to save lives. Unlike ammunition, it cannot be saved indefinitely. Because the blood cells are only good for a 21 day period, a continuous supply is needed.

   k. The blood you give may save a life.

   l. STOP ZD, (Zero Donors)

   m. Your blood donation is life insurance.

   n. A white-uniformed medic watches a blue-green vein swell and stand out on the arm of a soldier lying on his back on a cot. The medic leans over the man and deftly inserts a sharp, hollow needle into the vein, securing it with adhesive tape. Dark red blood begins to flow into the transparent tubing connected to the hollow needle. The soldier with the needle in his arm is not sick.

Attachment 2-2.

On the contrary, he's in the best of health, and he's "sharing his health" so that others may live. He's a Blood Donor.....

o. You know... giving blood is an easy thing. It is also about the most human thing you can do. Our modern medical skills can develop fine drugs create articles of life saving importance, teach operating techiques....just about anyting....but, the medical laboratory has never been able to make blood in a test tube. This is one thing that must be the gift of one man to another. Your gift is needed tody.... A visit to the Blood Center could save somebody's life... Maybe even yours.

p. What is a human life worth to you? Would you let an American fighting man die, when only a small effort on your part could save his life? Of course you would't.....So do something about it now... Visit your Unit Blood Collection Point during this month's drive and donate. Many times one pint can mean the difference between a wounded man's recovery.....and his death.

Attachment 2-2. Continued

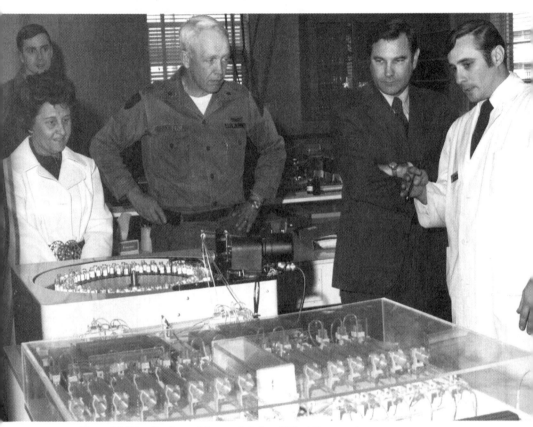

Figure 3-1. Brigadier General George S. Patton IV, Post Commander, Ft Knox, visiting the Blood Bank Center in 1972. Photograph from Camp Memorial Blood Center closure files. Courtesy of the Army Blood Program Office.

CHAPTER THREE

Commitment to Quality and Safety: 1970s

As the Vietnam War slowly came to a close in the early 1970s, Army blood bank officers focused on lessons learned over the past decade to lay the foundation for a formal Army blood program. It was also a time when leaders took steps to show the program's commitment to quality and safety. The program began preparation for individual blood donor centers to become accredited by the AABB (formerly known as the American Association of Blood Banks) and licensed by the Food and Drug Administration (FDA).

POST-VIETNAM WAR

As the US blood industry entered a new decade, it faced significant problems. It did not have a good system for ensuring a sufficient and safe blood supply and paid donors were the largest source of donations. President Richard Nixon signed Proclamation 3952, National Blood Donor Month, on December 31, 1969 (Exhibit 3-1).[1] He noted that the number of voluntary blood donors continued to grow, thanked donors for their generosity, and encouraged others to become voluntary donors. The proclamation designated January 1970 as National Blood Donor Month.[1] Unfortunately, industry concerns persisted because paid donors continued to be in the majority. This largely contributed to—among other things—significant inventory shortages across the country and a large number of transfusion-associated hepatitis cases. On March 2, 1972, as part of his special message to Congress on healthcare, President Nixon stated:

> Blood is a unique national resource. An adequate system for collecting and delivering blood at its time and place of need can save many lives. Yet we do not have a nationwide system to meet this need and we need to draw upon the skills of modern management and technology to develop

one. I have therefore directed the Department of Health, Education and Welfare to make an intensive study and to recommend to me as soon as possible a plan for developing a safe, fast and efficient nationwide blood collection system.[1]

This proclamation resulted in the development of the National Blood Policy, which contained 10 goals that led to an all-volunteer blood donation system and the creation of the American Blood Commission. The American Blood Commission would serve as the single entity for civilian (private sector) blood center accountability. Casper Weinberger, secretary of the Department of Health, Education, and Welfare, directed facilities to develop implementation plans for their organization in July 1973.[2] In 1974, President Nixon reiterated the importance of volunteer blood donation (Exhibit 3-2). Over the next few years, some paid donors were still used by facilities for various reasons. Therefore, in 1978 the FDA required blood banks to label their blood products as originating from either a paid or volunteer donor.[3]

In the 1970s, new blood program officers began to make their mark on the Army Blood Program. In early 1973, the first continental United States (CONUS) medical facility to establish a local frozen red blood cell program was Walter Reed Army Medical Center (WRAMC), under the leadership of Major John Radcliffe (US Army Blood Bank Fellowship [BBF] class of '68–69). This was followed 6 months later by Brooke Army Medical Center (BAMC), under the leadership of Major James Spiker, chief of the blood bank and donor center at Ft Sam Houston. Prior to this, frozen blood was thawed and transfused to patients for only a brief time during the Vietnam War. Now, the larger CONUS hospitals were starting the program. They used deglycerolized red cells, providing better clinical outcomes for patients with antibodies to rare antigens and preventing febrile transfusion reactions. The Navy established its own frozen blood program and was briefly involved in using deglycerolized red cells during the early part of the Vietnam War, but later used these products only for research. Since Navy research was already well under way, the Army agreed to let the Navy continue its focus on research while the Army would focus primarily on clinical advances so as not to duplicate efforts.

During his tenure at BAMC, Major Spiker continued his influence by expanding the array of available blood components at BAMC by routinely making platelet concentrates from whole blood donations. He also initiated a salvage plasma program for the Army and initiated shipments of excess red blood cells received from the Armed Services Whole Blood Processing Laboratory for input into the AABB clearinghouse exchange system for military credits, according to Colonel (Retired) Anthony Polk's email dated August 2010.

Proclamation 3952
NATIONAL BLOOD DONOR MONTH
By the President of the United States of America
December 31, 1969
A Proclamation

Genuine concern for his fellowman has always distinguished the American citizen. That concern finds daily expression in countless acts of voluntary service to the less fortunate, the sick, and the injured.

No manifestation of this generosity of spirit is more expressive, and no gift more priceless in time of personal crisis, than the donation of one's blood. The voluntary blood donor truly gives life itself.

Mobilized through the American Red Cross and the American Association of Blood Banks, and encouraged by modern medical techniques for simple and efficient collection and use of blood and its therapeutic components, the ranks of the voluntary blood donor have continued to grow and to make unparalleled contributions to the health of our people.

With the advent of the New Year, it is appropriate and timely to pay high tribute to our Nation's voluntary blood donors for their generosity and to encourage more people—both women and men, and both the younger and the older—to join their worthy ranks by providing a steady and increasing supply of blood during each month of the year ahead.

To this end, the Congress by Senate Joint Resolution 154 has requested the President to issue a proclamation designating the month of January 1970 as National Blood Donor Month.

83 Stat. 804.

NOW, THEREFORE, I, RICHARD NIXON, President of the United States of America, do hereby designate the month of January 1970 as National Blood Donor Month. I call upon the public media, the blood-banking and medical and health facilities of our country, and the public at large to pay special tribute and honor during that month to the voluntary blood donor and to encourage, by all appropriate means, increasing numbers of people to be voluntary blood donors.

IN WITNESS WHEREOF, I have hereunto set my hand this thirty-first day of December, in the year of our Lord nineteen hundred and sixty-nine, and of the Independence of the United States of America the one hundred and ninety-fourth.

Richard Nixon

Exhibit 3-1. Presidential proclamation designating National Blood Donor Month. Source: 3 CFR, 1970 Comp.

THE WHITE HOUSE
WASHINGTON

National Volunteer Blood Donor Month

January, 1974

Volunteer blood donation is recognized as one of the noblest and most vital gifts. There is no substitute for blood. There is no substitute for the voluntary donor.

During this special observance, I encourage all Americans to follow the inspiring example of those who have freely given blood to save another life. There is no better way than this to demonstrate true human compassion and generosity.

Richard Nixon

Exhibit 3-2. Letter signed by President Nixon in January 1974 recognizing volunteer blood donors and the importance of the gift of blood. Courtesy of the Army Blood Program Office.

Blood banking operations also contributed to the biological body of knowledge. In 1972, a very rare blood sample came through the BAMC blood bank. The sample turned out to be from the 11th Rh Null individual reported in the world, an Army medic stationed at Ft Sam Houston. With further investigation and testing, the medic's sister was also found to be Rh Null. This rarest of blood types lacks the A, B, and even the O antigen structures and can be a lifesaver for certain individuals.

Lieutenant Colonel Frank Camp established a blood donor center, called the Blood Bank Center, in 1971. Brigadier General George S. Patton IV showed his interest by visiting the center and meeting the staff (Figure 3-1). This was one of many expansion projects of the blood program at Ft Knox, which also had programs in operations, training, and blood research. Research projects ranged from expediting blood grouping by automation to red cell and platelet metabolism during storage.[4]

As another means to improve upon the safety of blood, Spectra Biologics and Abbott Laboratories developed and were licensed to manufacture hepatitis-associated antibody (anti-Australia antigen) as a test for hepatitis B in 1971 (Exhibit 3-3). Abbott's methodology was solid-phase radioimmunoassay, which was now the second test to screen for infectious diseases known to be transmitted by blood transfusions.[5] Donor centers then began routine screening of donors of whole blood and plasma.

On June 16, 1972, Department of Defense Directive 6480.5, *Military Blood Program,* was issued (Attachment 3-1). This new document rescinded the 1962 directive, and provided additional and more specific responsibilities.[6] It also recognized the agency's name change from the Military Blood Program Agency to the Military Blood Program Office (MBPO). It would be another 8 years before the Army established a specific regulation to identify the mission and functions of the MBPO.

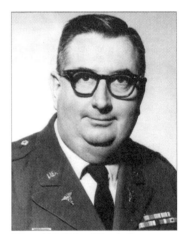

Figure 3-2. Colonel Frank Camp Jr. 1973. Photograph from Camp Memorial Blood Center closure files. Courtesy of the Army Blood Program Office.

The following year, in 1973, Colonel Frank Camp (Figure 3-2), Colonel Nicholas Conte, and Lieutenant Colonel Jerry Brewer (BBF class of '65–66) published *Military Blood Banking 1941–1973: Lessons Learned Applicable to Civil Disasters and Other Considerations.*[4] The primary purpose of this monograph was

C O P Y

U. S. DEPARTMENT OF
HEALTH, EDUCATION, AND WELFARE
Public Health Service
National Institutes of Health
Division of Biologics Standards
Bethesda, Maryland 20014
April 13, 1971

TO : All Licensed Manufacturers

FROM : Assistant Director, Division of Biologics Standards

SUBJECT: Screening of Blood for the Presence of Australia Antigen

On February 19, 1971, Spectra Biologicals and on March 15, 1971, Abbott Laboratories were licensed to manufacture Hepatitis Associated Antibody (Anti-Australia Antigen). Other companies are in the process of qualifying for licensure. The amount of this reagent available for general use is increasing but not yet sufficient for use by all licensed establishments to screen blood donors. Until such time as supplies are adequate so that screening of all blood donors can be required, we recommend that routine screening of donors of Whole Blood (Human) be instituted by each blood bank at the earliest opportunity. Blood that shows a positive reaction should be quarantined and must not be issued for transfusion or the preparation of components or fractions. As supplies of reagents increase, donors of plasma for fractionation should similarly be tested and positive reactors should be discarded. It is the intention of this Division to require this procedure at the earliest possible date for all blood collected under U. S. license and in the case of all plasma collected for fractionation.

Please inform this Division when you expect such testing to become routine in your establishment.

Sincerely yours,

Sam T. Gibson, M. D.

Exhibit 3-3. Notification from Public Health Service, National Institutes of Health, that Abbott Laboratories and Spectra Biologicals received licenses to manufacture Hepatitis Associated Antibody (Anti-Australia Antigen). April 13, 1971. Courtesy of the Armed Services Blood Program Office.

to apply lessons learned from the military blood program in previous combat operations to the medical management of small to medium mass casualties at US civilian medical centers.

In one of the earliest attempts to automate blood bank information, Major John Radcliff and Lieutenant Colonel Michael Hannagan, Medical Corps, developed a storage and retrieval system while in charge of the blood bank at WRAMC in 1973. This new system allowed the staff to track units of blood that came into the facility and were transfused into patients.[7]

The US blood industry continued to move forward on blood research and development. In 1979 citrate phosphate dextrose adenine, or CPDA-1, was introduced as a new anticoagulant and extended the shelf life of red blood cells from 21 to 35 days. The expansion of the shelf life made blood inventory management easier.

FOUNDATIONS OF THE MODERN ARMY BLOOD PROGRAM

The foundations of the modern Army Blood Program began on April 1, 1973, when the Army activated the US Army Health Services Command (HSC) at San Antonio, Texas, with Major General Spurgeon Neel as the first commander. Pursuant to the Department of the Army General Order Number 7 dated February 26, 1973,[8] and as part of a reorganization of the Army Medical Department, the newly established organization assumed command and control of most military treatment facilities within CONUS, Alaska, Hawaii, and Panama, and reported directly to the chief of staff of the US Army. This allowed the Office of The Surgeon General (OTSG), whose transfusion branch had previously worked with the blood research program at the Army Medical School, to focus more on staff and technical supervisory duties as the principal advisor to the chief of staff of the Army on health and medical issues.[8]

HSC was the major command that oversaw the Army Blood Program within CONUS. Overseas commands established their own blood programs, similar to the structure in CONUS. During this period, OTSG retained its overall control of the Army Blood Program, but allowed HSC considerable freedom (Figure 3-3). Blood banks at the HSC regional medical centers became regional coordinators and received clearinghouse accreditation by the AABB. Clearinghouse accreditation enabled regional coordinators to transfer blood between military and civilian facilities.[9]

Lieutenant Colonel James Spiker (Figure 3-4) was the first HSC clinical laboratory and blood bank consultant, serving from 1974 to 1979. One of Lieutenant Colonel Spiker's key accomplishments was the inclusion of Army

```
                    ┌─────────────────────────┐
                    │  ARMY SURGEON GENERAL   │
                    └─────────────────────────┘
                           │           │
              ┌────────────┘           └────────────┐
              ▼                                     ▼
    ┌───────────────────┐               ┌───────────────────────────┐
    │ OVERSEAS COMMANDS │               │ HEADQUARTERS HSC (CONUS)  │
    └───────────────────┘               └───────────────────────────┘

    ┌───────────────────┐               ┌───────────────────────────┐
    │  COMMAND SURGEON  │               │   REGIONAL COORDINATOR    │
    └───────────────────┘               └───────────────────────────┘

    ┌───────────────────┐               ┌───────────────────────────┐
    │ BLOOD DONOR CENTER*│              │   BLOOD DONOR CENTER*     │
    │  Operated by MTF  │               │      Operated by MTF      │
    └───────────────────┘               └───────────────────────────┘
```

*Installation Commanders (Supply Donors)

Figure 3-3. Relationships in the Army Blood Program April 1, 1973 to June 30, 1975, from US Army Health Services Command. Reproduced from *US Army Health Services Command*. Annual Historical Review April 1, 1973, to June 30, 1975. Ft Sam Houston, TX: HSC; 1978: 232.

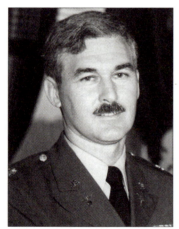

Figure 3-4. Lieutenant Colonel James Spiker, Health Services Command Clinical Lab/Blood Bank Consultant. Courtesy of Colonel (Ret) James Spiker Jr.

blood donor centers in HSC Mobilization Exercise 1978, also known as "Exercise Nifty Nugget." In this "real world" exercise, 10 donor centers collected whole blood from actual donors, up to 50 units per day of the exercise, and then shipped the unprocessed blood to the blood bank center at Ft Knox.[10] One of the lessons learned from this exercise was that—at a minimum—a second blood bank center was needed in the Army to keep up with component requirements, which was the impetus for constructing the Blood Bank Center at Ft Hood[11] (Figures 3-5 and 3-6). Lieutenant Colonel Spiker was followed by Lieutenant Colonel Robert Usry (Figure 3-7) (BBF class of '72–73), Lieutenant Colonel Gerald Jacobs (Figure 3-8), and Colonel Richard Platte (Figure 3-9) (BBF class of '84–85).

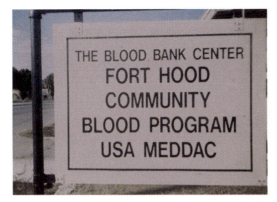

Figure 3-5. [Top] Sign in front of The Blood Bank Center (TBBC) Ft Hood, Texas. Courtesy of Colonel (Ret) Anthony Polk.

Figure 3-6. [Bottom] The original blood donor center building on Ft Hood. Captain Anthony Polk's teenage sons painted the building with the light green paint provided by the facility engineers. Courtesy of Colonel (Ret) Anthony Polk.

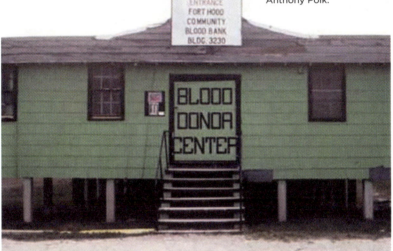

ACCREDITATION AND LICENSURE

The blood donor centers and hospital-based transfusion services began to formalize as a program under the HSC by 1974. Coordination and organization of the various blood donor centers and other blood-related operations were underway worldwide. The jurisdiction of the US Army Medical Research Laboratory's blood donor center at Ft Knox changed from OTSG to HSC in July 1974.[8] As the first HSC laboratory and blood bank consultant, Spiker focused on FDA licensure. HSC blood banks could also receive AABB accreditation, when geographical location required it, such as at overseas locations. Hospital transfusions services were also to be accredited by the AABB. Over the next year and a half, Lieutenant Colonel Spiker made tremendous progress as other

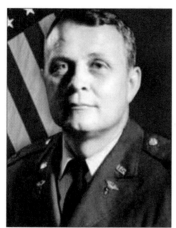

Figure 3-7. Lieutenant Colonel Robert Usry. Courtesy of Mr. Bill Turcan, US Army Blood Bank Fellowship.

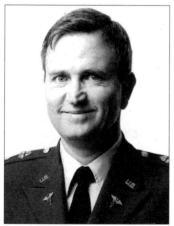

Figure 3-8. Lieutenant Colonel Gerald Jacobs. Courtesy of Lieutenant Colonel (Ret) Gerald Jacobs.

facilities obtained FDA licensure and AABB accreditation. By mid-1975, 85% of blood donor centers and transfusion services had received accreditation, and seven of eight medical centers served as clearinghouses in the national program. Additionally, all eight medical centers had submitted their applications for FDA licensure and were scheduled for inspection by the end of the year. In preparation, Lieutenant Colonel Spiker coordinated and performed pre-inspection consultations with all HSC sites.[9]

On September 26, 1974, key leadership from the MBPO, the service blood programs, and the FDA met to discuss inspection and licensure procedures for the military blood banks. Attending from the FDA were Ms. Madge Crouch, Dr. Lou Barker, and Mr. Scheno. The military was represented by Colonel Hal Etter from the MBPO; Colonel Charles Angel, OTSG lab consultant; Lieutenant Colonel Turman Allen from WRAMC; Lieutenant Commander Jason Wilson and Chief Petty Officer Ralph Hanson from Navy Bureau of Medicine and Surgery; and Major Hubert Wrenn from the Air Force surgeon general's office, according to Kathleen Elder's email dated January 2012. Colonel Angel was a biochemist and wanted an Army blood bank officer to attend this meeting. Unfortunately, Lieutenant Colonel Spiker was unable to make the trip to Washington, DC, so Lieutenant Colonel Allen, the blood bank officer at WRAMC, represented Spiker, according to his own email dated June 2014.

After discussion, the following agreements were made according to Ms. Kathleen Elder's email, dated February 2012:

- A prelicensure inspection schedule would be announced so that key personnel at the activity would be present.

- All correspondence to the FDA would emanate from the licensee (offices of the surgeon general), not from the individual facilities or lower echelon commands.[9]
- Upon completion of the inspection, an exit interview would be held with the facility commander or their designated representative, and the inspector's findings would be verbally presented. No written report would be furnished at the time.
- The three services would endeavor to submit initial licensure applications by January 1, 1975. At the time, the Army planned to submit applications for eight installations, the Navy planned for five installations, and the Air Force planned for seven installations.
- It was anticipated that prelicensure inspections would be held 60 to 90 days following application submissions. Licensing procedures were expected to be completed by July 1, 1975.
- It was agreed that the Armed Services Whole Blood Processing Laboratory would be licensed under the Air Force.

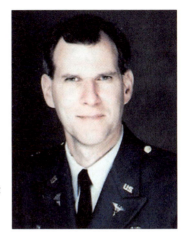

Figure 3-9. Colonel Richard Platte. Courtesy of Colonel (Ret) Richard Platte.

Early in the summer of 1974, the Department of Defense entered into an agreement with the FDA to establish a uniform policy on the voluntary licensure of military blood banks according to the Public Health Service Act, without compromising the unique nature and capabilities of the military blood system (FDA-MOU 74-12, Attachment 3-2).

On March 7, 1975, BAMC became the first Army facility to receive its FDA license (Figure 3-10). BAMC's license submission was approved for whole blood, red blood cells, and single-donor plasma. This license allowed the facility to collect, manufacture, and exchange these blood products with other facilities, both military and civilian, by adhering to the requirements of the Public Health Service Act and the Federal Food, Drug, and Cosmetic Act.[12] Just a few months later, on June 19, WRAMC received its FDA license.

On September 25, 1975, five more blood donor centers were added to the Army's blood establishment license (FDA license 611):

- Fitzsimons Army Medical Center
- William Beaumont Army Medical Center
- Eisenhower Army Medical Center
- Tripler Army Medical Center
- Madigan Army Medical Center

The donor centers were approved to manufacture whole blood using acid-citrate-dextrose and citrate-phosphate-dextrose (CPD), anticoagulants, and red blood cells. Single donor and fresh frozen plasma were approved for all locations except Fitzsimons. BAMC's license was expanded to cover cryoprecipitated antihemophilic factor and whole blood modified, cryoprecipitate removed. On June 21, 1976, the Army Medical Department activities at Ft Knox were added to the Department of the Army's FDA 611 license, according to Kathleen Elder's email dated January 2012. Letterman Army Hospital was the lone medical center not licensed.[8]

A change in the oversight of the Army Blood Program occurred in 1979. The HSC clinical laboratory and blood bank consultant was put in charge of operations, while the blood bank officer at OTSG took charge of policy. This division of responsibilities continued until 1994, when the Army Blood Program went through another extensive restructuring according to Colonel (Retired) Anthony Polk's email dated August 2010.

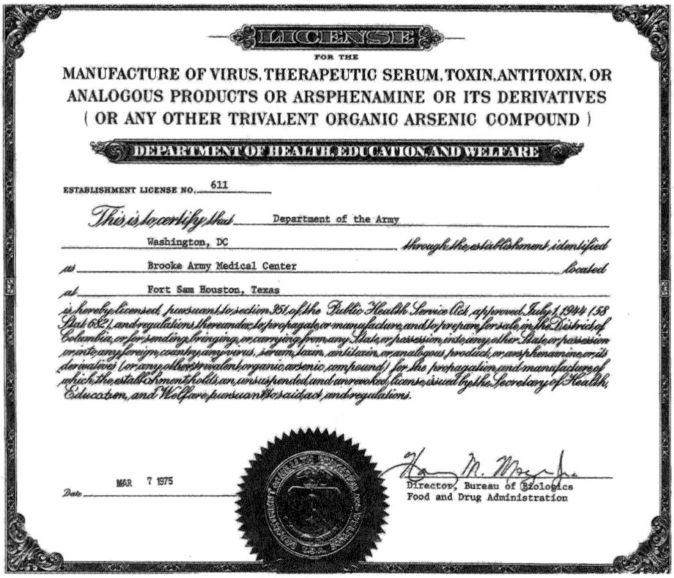

LICENSE

FOR THE

MANUFACTURE OF VIRUS, THERAPEUTIC SERUM, TOXIN, ANTITOXIN, OR ANALOGOUS PRODUCTS OR ARSPHENAMINE OR ITS DERIVATIVES (OR ANY OTHER TRIVALENT ORGANIC ARSENIC COMPOUND)

DEPARTMENT OF HEALTH, EDUCATION, AND WELFARE

ESTABLISHMENT LICENSE NO. 611

This is to certify that Department of the Army Washington, DC through the establishment identified as Brooke Army Medical Center located at Fort Sam Houston, Texas is hereby licensed, pursuant to section 351 of the Public Health Service Act, approved July 1, 1944 (58 Stat. 682), and regulations thereunder, to propagate or manufacture, and to prepare for sale in the District of Columbia, or for sending, bringing, or carrying from any State or possession into any other State or possession or into any foreign country any virus, serum, toxin, antitoxin, or analogous product, or arsphenamine or its derivatives (or any other trivalent organic arsenic compound) for the propagation and manufacture of which the establishment holds an unsuspended and unrevoked license, issued by the Secretary of Health, Education, and Welfare pursuant to said act and regulations.

Date MAR 7 1975

Director, Bureau of Biologics
Food and Drug Administration

Figure 3-10. BAMC's FDA license, March 7, 1975.

SUMMARY

Throughout the 1970s, the Army Blood Program, in many ways, followed with the rest of the US blood industry, showing its commitment to safety and quality by collecting blood from volunteer donors, and pursuing FDA licensure and AABB accreditation. Additionally, unlike our civilian counterparts, the Army also continued improving readiness through expanded use of frozen red blood cells and the establishment of another Blood Bank Center. The efforts on both of these fronts led the Army to become a premier blood program.

REFERENCES

1. Nixon R. Proclamation 3952—National Blood Donor Month. December 31, 1969. Online by Gerhard Peters and John T. Woolley, The American Presidency Project. http://www.presidency.ucsb.edu/ws/?pid=23771. Accessed June 1, 2016.
2. US National Library of Medicine. US Department of Health Education and Welfare, national blood policy records, 1969–1981. http://oculus.nlm.nih.gov/cgi/f/findaid/findaid-idx?c=nlmfindaid;cc=nlmfindaid;view=reslist;subview=standard;didno=hew393;focusrgn=bioghist;byte=16251560. Updated June 16, 2014. Accessed June 1, 2016.
3. Henry JB, Hubbel RC. Blood policy and strategy: The American Blood Commission and the nation's blood resource. *Hum Pathol.* 1980;11(1):1–3.
4. Camp FR, Conte N, Brewer JR. *Military Blood Banking 1941–1973–Lessons Learned Applicable to Civil Disasters and Other Considerations.* Fort Knox, KY: US Army Medical Research Laboratory, Blood Bank Center; 1973.
5. US Department of Health, Education, and Welfare. *Screening of Blood for the Presence of Australia Antigen.* Bethesda, MD: Public Health Services, National Institutes of Health. Letter, April 13, 1971.
6. US Department of Defense. *Military Blood Program.* Washington, DC: DoD; 1972. DoD Directive 6480.5.
7. Ginn RVN. *The History of the US Army Medical Service Corps.* Washington, DC: DA, Office of The Surgeon General and Center of Military History; 1997.
8. US Department of the Army. *Annual Report of the Surgeon General, United States Army 1972/73–1974/75.* Washington, DC: DA, Office of The Surgeon General; 1975.
9. US Department of the Army. *US Army Health Service Command Annual Historical Review, 1 April 1973 to 30 June 1975.* Washington, DC: DA; 1978. http://cdm15290.contentdm.oclc.org/cdm/singleitem/collection/p16379coll8/id/3/rec/5. Accessed June 1, 2016.
10. US Department of the Army. *HSC Mobilization Exercise 78—Annex H (Blood Program).* Fort Sam Houston, TX: DA, Health Services Command; 1978.
11. US Department of the Army. *Staff Visit to Review Clinical Laboratory Operations and Observe Joint Fort Hood/BAMC Blood Donor Operations.* Fort Sam Houston, TX: DA, Health Services Command. Staffing packet, June 5, 1979.
12. 42 USCA §262. *The Public Health and Welfare.* Washington, DC. 1938.

June 16, 1972
NUMBER 6480.5

ASD(H&E)

Department of Defense Directive

SUBJECT Military Blood Program

Refs: (a) DoD Directive 6480.5, "Department of Defense Blood Program," May 15, 1962 (hereby cancelled)
(b) Defense Mobilization Order 8540.2, "Policy Guidance for a National Emergency Blood Program
(c) DoD Directive 5000.19, "Policies for the Management and Control of DoD Information Requirements," June 2, 1971

I. PURPOSE

A. This Directive (1) delineates the scope of the military blood program; (2) establishes the Military Blood Program Office (MBPO) to coordinate the blood programs of the Military Departments; (3) defines the responsibilities of the Military Departments for the support of the Department of Defense Military Blood Program; and (4) assigns certain responsibilities for the support of the Military Blood Program.

B. The program is designed to meet the needs for blood and blood components of all patients receiving medical care in military medical treatment facilities and to respond to selected emergency civilian situations upon approval by appropriate authority.

II. CANCELLATION

Reference (a) is hereby superseded and cancelled.

III. APPLICABILITY AND SCOPE

A. The provisions of this Directive apply to the Military Departments, Organization of the Joint Chiefs of Staff, and the Unified and Specified Commands.

B. The DoD Military Blood Program encompasses the blood program of the organizations listed in A., above, and the Military Blood Program Office. It includes:

1. The collection (at military installations), processing,

Attachment 3-1.

distribution and use of whole blood and its fractions by military hospitals on a local or regional basis according to the policies of the respective Military Departments;

2. The procurement of whole blood and blood components, for military use, from sources outside the Department of Defense;

3. The maintenance and implementation (by ASD(H&E), MBPO and the Military Departments) of plans to provide for the collection, processing and distribution of whole blood and its fractions to the Armed Forces, worldwide, for day-to-day operations and under all degrees of emergency;

4. The provision and maintenance of a source of trained personnel, facilities, and supplies and equipment, adequate to meet initial emergency requirements; and

5. A research and development program devoted to progress and improvement in the areas of blood, blood derivatives, and plasma volume expanders, and the techniques, facilities and materiel related thereto.

IV. POLICY

A. The Military Departments will maintain separate Military Blood Programs to meet the overall whole blood and blood component requirements of all patients receiving medical care in military medical treatment facilities.

B. Appropriate efforts will be made to minimize any adverse impact on blood programs of civilian communities adjacent to military installations. All blood collections by the Military Departments will be limited to military installations. Accordingly, collections will be restricted to military personnel, their dependents, and civilian personnel on such military installations.

C. The Military Departments will take appropriate steps to insure proper management of whole blood, its components and available donor resources.

V. MILITARY BLOOD PROGRAM OFFICE

A. Organization. There is hereby established the Military Blood Procurement Office to coordinate the blood programs of the Military Departments.

1. The MBPO shall consist of three medical department officers in the grade of O-4 or above, one from each of the Military Departments.

Attachment 3-1. Continued

6480.5
June 16, 72

2. A medical department officer, selected by agreement among the Surgeons General of the Army, Navy and Air Force with the concurrence of ASD(H&E), will be appointed as Director of the Military Blood Program Office. The other members will be designated as deputy directors.

3. Each member shall represent his Department and should have direct access to his Surgeon General.

B. Functions. The MBPO will perform the following functions:

1. Monitor the implementation of the Military Blood Program policy guidance established by the Assistant Secretary of Defense (Health and Environment).

2. Maintain and disseminate plans for coordinating the collection, processing, distribution, and management of blood and blood components necessary to meet the requirements of the Military Departments.

3. Coordinate the plans, policies and procedures as outlined in paragraph 2 above with the Military Departments, and Unified and Specified Commands.

4. Coordinate Military Blood Program plans and actions which have military operational implications with the Joint Chiefs of Staff.

5. Prescribe information requirements as necessary to insure program effectiveness. Such information requirements will be consistent with the policies prescribed in reference (c).

6. Provide technical and professional guidance to the Defense Supply Agency on the procurement of whole blood and blood components, when required, and on mobilization and industrial mobilization requirements for natural and synthetic plasma expanders.

7. Provide direct liaison with other Government and civilian agencies having an interest in blood and related items.

8. Develop, recommend and monitor policies (fully coordinated with the Military Departments) on:

   (a) The collection, procurement, processing, storage, distribution, and management of whole blood.

   (b) The acceptability, distribution, and use of blood components and synthetic or other non-human plasma volume expanders.

9. Obtain and maintain, on a continuing basis, emergency and mobilization military requirements of whole blood from the Military Departments and Unified and Specified Commands, as appropriate; and determine net DoD requirements.

10. Designate, and if necessary, prepare approved written guides relating to all phases of blood banking procedures to be used as minimum standards by the military services.

11. Receive and take appropriate action on overseas originated requests from theater commanders for whole blood and blood components, and according to the policies of the Military Department involved, receive and take appropriate action on CONUS originated requirements for whole blood and components which exceed departmental resources.

12. Request, when authorized by the Assistant Secretary of Defense (Health and Environment), that the Defense Supply Agency activate the standby contracts for procurement of blood from civilian sources whenever the military requirements exceed the internal blood collection and processing capabilities of the Military Departments.

13. Coordinate with the Defense Medical Materiel Board on essential characteristics of materiel associated with military blood banking.

14. Coordinate research and development requirements of the DoD Blood Program, conveying these requirements through ASD(H&E) to DDR&E.

15. Coordinate technical aspects of blood research programs when requested by DDR&E.

C. Support. Administrative support for the MBPO will be provided as outlined in VI.C.1, below.

VI. RESPONSIBILITIES

A. The Assistant Secretary of Defense (Health and Environment) is responsible for providing overall policy guidance on the DoD Military Blood Program, and for coordinating it with the National Emergency Blood Program, when required.

B. The Director, Defense Research and Engineering is responsible for coordinating and issuing policy guidance on military department research and development projects related to the Military Blood Program.

Attachment 3-1. Continued

6480.6
Jun 16, 72

C. The Secretary of the Army, or his designee, in support of the DoD Military Blood Program will:

1. Maintain operational control of the MBPO and provide administrative support for its internal administration and operation. (The term "Administrative support" as used in this Directive includes civilian personnel requirements, civilian personnel and security administration, inspection, space, facilities, supplies, and other administrative provisions and services as required to assure that the responsibilities of the MBPO can be properly discharged.)

2. Program, budget, and finance all costs of operations of the MBPO and its staff, except the pay, allowances, and PCS travel of military personnel members and assigned staff which are the responsibility of the Military Department providing the military personnel.

3. Fund for blood procurement from civilian sources including the costs of transportation to the appropriate Armed Services Whole Blood Processing Laboratory (ASWBPL) when overall military requirements exceed the organic capability of the military services. However, nothing in this or any other section of this Directive shall preclude a service from obtaining local purchases of blood in any emergency where time or other considerations make such purchase desirable.

D. The Secretary of the Air Force, or his designee, will:

1. Designate ASWBPL at CONUS air terminals for whole blood shipments from CONUS.

2. Coordinate the joint staffing of the designated ASWBPL's by medical personnel of the Army, Navy and Air Force in accordance with staffing criteria concurred in by the providing services.

3. Provide administrative support for the designated ASWBPL's.

4. Program, budget and finance all costs of maintenance and operations of the ASWBPL's at CONUS air terminals and the staffs, except the pay, allowances, and PCS travel, of military personnel assigned to the Laboratories. These latter costs are the responsibility of the Military Department providing the military personnel.

5. Maintain the ASWBPL's in a standby status, when not activated to support day-to-day operations, in order that they will be capable of activation and functional operation within 7 days on request of the Military Blood Program Office.

5

Attachment 3-1. Continued

6. Obtain concurrence of the ASD(H&E) through the MBPO prior to closing or deactivating an ASWBPL operating in accordance with this Directive.

7. Transport whole blood from an ASWBPL at CONUS air terminals to the destination designated by the Military Blood Program Office. In the event it becomes necessary to relocate a CONUS air terminal or ASWBPL or to establish a Whole Blood Transshipment Center on another Military Airlift Command designated location, the Air Force is responsible for transportation of the whole blood and blood components from such location to the destination designated by the Military Blood Program Office.

E. The Secretaries of the Army, Navy and Air Force, and the Commanders of Unified and Specified Commands will:

1. Maintain internal departmental and command blood programs emphasizing the importance of command leadership in motivating personnel to support the Military Blood Program. The blood programs shall provide for the collection of whole blood and blood components at military installations; for processing and distributing these products to meet (a) normal departmental or command requirements, (b) (within their capabilities) requirements generated by military operations as well as local, regional, or national emergencies, and (c) providing donor support to other service blood programs provided such support does not degrade the capability to support command or departmental blood programs.

2. Insure that their respective blood programs reflect the policies established herein, and the guidance developed and promulgated by the ASD(H&E).

3. Insure that their blood programs can be readily expanded to satisfy requirements for whole blood and blood components.

4. Submit requirements and reporting capabilities as requested, to the Military Blood Program Office.

5. Insure that additional facilities and augmentation personnel required to support the Military Blood Program incident to any emergency situation are included in Program Change Requests submitted by the Military Departments.

6. Fund for the transportation of whole blood and incidental expenses associated with the delivery of whole blood to the first CONUS destination as designated by the MBPO.

Attachment 3-1. Continued

```
                                                    6480.5
                                                    Jun 16, 72
```

F. The Director, Defense Supply Agency, is responsible for the procurement and stockpiling of plasma expanders, both natural and synthetic, and other blood products in accordance with guidance provided the Military Blood Procurement Office and the Defense Medical Materiel Board. He is also responsible for annually reviewing standard contract agreements between the Military Blood Procurement Office and the American Red Cross and American Association of Blood Banks.

G. The Director, Military Blood Program Office is responsible for executing the functions cited in VI.C., 1-15. These responsibilities shall be met by direct liaison and coordination with military and governmental agencies cited in this Directive.

VII. EFFECTIVE DATE AND IMPLEMENTATION

This Directive is effective immediately. Within ninety days of receipt of this Directive (1) the Secretaries of the Army, Navy and Air Force shall develop such implementing instructions as are appropriate to their departments and (2) the Secretary of the Army shall develop in collaboration with the Secretaries of the Navy and Air Force, implementing instructions for the joint aspects of the Directive.

Kenneth Rush
Deputy Secretary of Defense

Attachment 3-1. Continued

FDA-MOU 74-12

MEMORANDUM OF UNDERSTANDING
BETWEEN THE
DEPARTMENT OF DEFENSE
AND THE
FOOD AND DRUG ADMINISTRATION

The Department of Defense (hereinafter called DOD) and the Food and Drug Administration of the Department of Health, Education, and Welfare (hereinafter called FDA) hereby jointly agree to the terms and conditions as described herein.

Purpose: To establish a uniform policy between the Department of Defense and the Food and Drug Administration relative to the voluntary licensure of military blood banks pursuant to Section 351 of the Public Health Service Act.

Background

Blood, blood components or derivatives, or analogous products applicable to the prevention, treatment, or cure of diseases or injuries of man (henceforth referred to as biological products) are potentially subject to the licensing provisions of Section 351 of the Public Health Service Act, which is enforced by the Bureau of Biologics of the Food and Drug Administration. These biological products are human "drugs" as that word is defined under the Federal Food, Drug, and Cosmetic Act, which is also enforced by the FDA. Biological products and the manufacture of such products are therefore subject to both Section 351 of the Public Health Service Act and the human drug provisions of the Federal Food, Drug, and Cosmetic Act.

The Department of Defense wishes to voluntarily avail itself of the licensing provisions of Section 351 of the Public Health Service Act, to enable the military to more freely and expeditiously exchange blood and blood components with civilian blood banks to more effectively utilize this vital national blood resource. The Food and Drug Administration, for its part, looks with favor upon the entrance and integration of certain aspects of the military blood system with that of the civilian system to move the nation's blood services complex more nearly towards one nationwide system with uniform standards of quality and safety.

Inasmuch as both the Food and Drug Administration and the Department of Defense recognize the unique nature and capabilities of the military blood banking system, and in recognition of their mutual recognition of the military need for flexibility to assure the common defense, a mechanism to implement the licensing provisions of Section 351 of the Public Health Service Act has been agreed upon which will adequately serve the public health goals of Section 351 without in any way compromising the military's capacity to respond effectively in meeting urgent military requirements.

Attachment 3-2.

FDA-MOU 74-12   Page 2

I. Substance of Agreement

The Food and Drug Administration and the Department of Defense agree that:

1. Upon application for FDA license, each military department volunteers to be licensed with respect to its military blood program.

2. Each military department will apply to the Food and Drug Administration for issue of a separate license. These licenses will be equivalent to those issued to civilian blood programs in accordance with Section 351 of the Public Health Service Act. Exceptions to the license not covered in this agreement will be coordinated by the military department concerned with the Food and Drug Administration.

3. Each military department will insure that its blood banking facilities will meet the standards prescribed and are operated in accordance with FDA blood banking regulations. Each military department on its own or in conjunction with other military departments, will provide for the inspection of its blood banks by qualified personnel to insure that the facilities are operated in accordance with FDA regulations. The inspections will use criteria equivalent to or exceeding those employed in the inspection of civilian blood banks.

4. FDA inspection of military blood banking facilities will be conducted as deemed necessary and will be coordinated with the licensee of each military department.

5. Discrepancies noted or deviations from the governing FDA regulations will be reported to the Surgeon General of the military service involved by the designated inspectors. Each Surgeon General shall be responsible for taking the corrective action necessary to insure compliance. Inspection reports will be available both to the Surgeons General and the FDA.

6. For national security, the Department of Defense must maintain a worldwide capability for medical care. The military departments during military operations, military and/or civilian emergencies may be required to deviate from the blood banking standards of the FDA. FDA will be made aware of the deviations from the FDA standards and their medical implications.

II. Name and Address of Participating Agencies

A. Department of Defense
   Washington, D. C. 20314

B. Food and Drug Administration
   5600 Fishers Lane
   Rockville, Maryland 20852

Attachment 3-2. Continued

FDA-MOU 74-12 Page 3

III. Liaison Officers

   A. Hal G. Etter, COL, BSC, USAF
      Director of Military Blood Program Office
      Office of the Surgeon General
      U. S. Army
      Department of Defense
      Washington, D. C. 20314
      Telephone: (202) 693-5575

   B. Mr. James O. Gesling
      Associate Director
      Bureau of Biologics, HFB-3
      Food and Drug Administration
      8800 Rockville Pike
      Bethesda, Maryland 20014
      Telephone: (301) 496-6807

IV. Period of Agreement

   This agreement, when accepted by both agencies, covers an indefinite period of time, and may be modified by mutual consent of both parties or terminated by either party upon a thirty (30) day advance written notice to the other.

APPROVED AND ACCEPTED FOR THE
DEPARTMENT OF DEFENSE

By _____
Title (Health and Environment)
   Actg Asst Secretary of Defense
Date   19 June 1974

APPROVED AND ACCEPTED FOR THE
FOOD AND DRUG ADMINISTRATION

By _____
Title Commissioner of Food & Drugs
Date   21 May 1974

Attachment 3-2. Continued

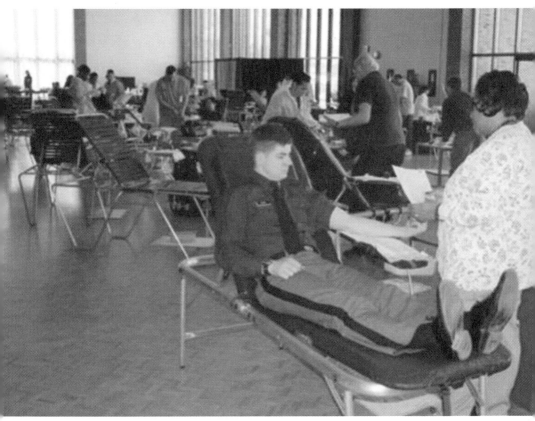

Figure 4-1. A cadet donates at the 2009 annual West Point blood drive. The history of the annual blood drive at the West Point Military Academy goes back many years. In addition to collecting needed units of blood, the blood drive exposed the cadets to the Armed Service Blood Program (ASBP) and its mission. As future commanders and leaders, they in turn, would emphasis the importance of the ASBP to their staff and soldiers. Courtesy of the Army Blood Program Office.

CHAPTER FOUR

Review, Refine, and Expand: 1980s

Much like the late 1970s, the 1980s allowed the Army Blood Program (ABP) opportunity to review doctrine and requirements, expand its capabilities, and work with the Food and Drug Administration (FDA) to ensure that all its blood donor centers were FDA licensed. On May 15, 1980, the Department of the Army issued Army Regulation 10-64, *Military Blood Program Office*.[1] This regulation established the mission and principal functions of the Military Blood Program Office (MBPO) (Attachment 4-1), as stated in Department of Defense (DoD) Directive 6480.5, June 16, 1972.[2] These efforts, both at the Army level and the Department of Defense level, would ensure a blood program that was capable of fully supporting future military operations with quality blood products and service.

CHANGE IN OPERATIONS

During the 1980s, a formal agreement between the ABP and the American Red Cross (ARC)—referred to as "Compass"—was in place across the United States. The program was in essence a credit and debit system of blood exchange in lieu of dollars passing hands. The Army was credited with blood units as they were collected on Army installations by ARC bloodmobiles, and Army hospitals could debit the Compass program on an as-needed basis against those credits. Chet Summerville was the ARC point of contact for the program. Eventually, Compass was scrapped because of resistance to the ARC collecting on military installations, especially where military donor centers routinely operated.

Major General Lewis Mologne, Walter Reed Army Medical Center's commander from 1983 to 1988, was a strong proponent and supporter of the ABP. However, he faced fierce competition with the ARC for military donors in

Figure 4-2. [Top] Another cadet donates at the 2009 West Point blood drive. There has been a long-standing competition among the cadets as to which class could donate the most units. Courtesy of the Army Blood Program Office.

Figure 4-3. [Bottom] Colonel Gary Norris recognizes a staff member at the West Point blood drive. Courtesy of the Army Blood Program Office.

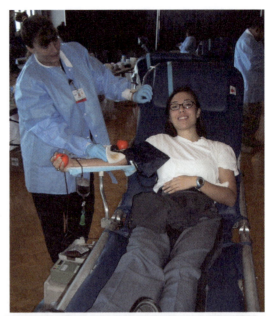

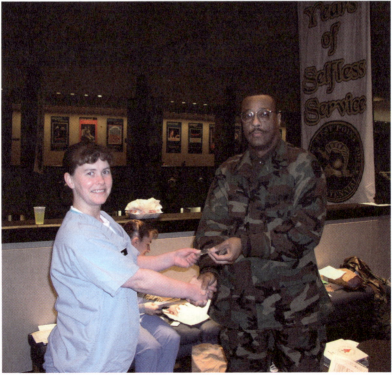

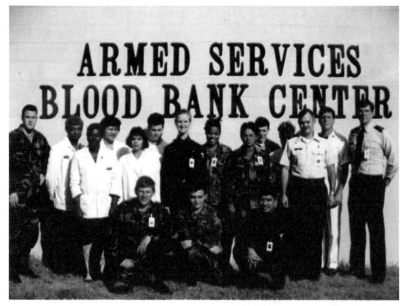

Figure 4-4. The Ft Ord Armed Services Blood Bank Center staff—the "original" ASBBC. Courtesy of Mr. David Hopper.

the Military District of Washington. A local supplement to AR 40-2, a regulation governing general administrative policies for all active Army military treatment facilities, said the ARC had the right to collect blood in the district to the exclusion of the Army. With the help of Major General Mologne, Lieutenant Colonel Richard Platte (US Army Blood Bank Fellowship [BBF] class of '84–85) rescinded the supplement, but it was still difficult for Walter Reed Army Medical Center to collect blood in Washington. However, Platte made inroads at Ft Belvoir, Virginia, and Ft Meade, Maryland. He also expanded collections at Aberdeen Proving Ground, Maryland, and continued active collections at the US Military Academy in West Point, New York (Figures 4-1 to 4-3), according to Colonel (Retired) into the 1990s Richard Platte's email dated November 2011.

The first tri-service blood donor center was established at Ft Ord, California, in 1985 (Figure 4-4). It was named the Armed Services Blood Bank Center, and it operated under the ABP's FDA blood establishment license and functioned as a regional blood supplier to military hospitals. Captain Gary Griffin (BBF class of '89–90) served as its first director.

As the first multi-service blood donor center, the Armed Services Blood Bank Center combined resources from smaller hospital-based donor centers of the Army, Navy, and Air Force in California in a single center to support all of the region's hospitals.[3]

REVIEW OF DOCTRINE AND REQUIREMENTS

The Military Field Medical Systems Standardization Steering Group directed the MBPO to conduct a zero-based analysis of program requirements for the mid- and long- term in 1983.[4] Captain James Bates, US Navy, director of the MBPO, initiated the analysis projecting out 20 years. Lieutenant Colonel Anthony Polk (Figure 4-5), who became MBPO director in 1984, believed that the three services managed good blood programs during peacetime, but the wartime capability—like most of the medical wartime capabilities since the end of the Vietnam War—was diminished or unknown. In 1985 Lieutenant Colonel Polk established the first formal blood coordinating committee, which produced formal minutes and an action list. Committee members were Lieutenant Colonel Polk; Colonel Jim Spiker, US Army; Captain Mike Ward, US Air Force; Lieutenant Commander Woody Woods, US Navy; and later Captain Jerry Baker, US Navy (Figure 4-6). From these meetings, the committee devised a plan that Lieutenant Colonel Polk named Military Blood Program (MBP) 2004. Two key recommendations noted in the 1995–2001 Medical Readiness Strategic Plan were the need for group O blood at echelon two and the use of frozen blood.[5] The assistant secretary of defense for health affairs (ASD[HA]) approved the report in May 1985. One month later, the MBPO convened a panel of experts to develop a plan and milestones for implementing MBP 2004's recommendations, according to Colonel (Retired) Anthony Polk's email communication, March 2014.

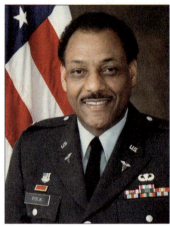

Figure 4-5. Colonel Anthony Polk. Courtesy of Colonel (Ret) Anthony Polk.

With the passing of the Goldwater-Nichols Department of Defense Reorganization Act of 1986, a tremendous change occurred in how the military participated in joint operations. Dr. William Mayer, the ASD(HA), placed an intense new focus on medical wartime capabilities. Within this focus, inadequate wartime blood capacity was labeled a "war stopper" according to Colonel (Retired) Anthony Polk in his email dated March 2014. Mayer created a Medical Readiness Directorate within Health Affairs and Lieutenant Colonel Polk reported directly to the general officer in charge of this directorate (initially Brigadier General France F. Jordan, followed by Major General Bill Winkler). While working with the Medical Readiness Directorate, Lieutenant Colonel Polk incorporated blood operations

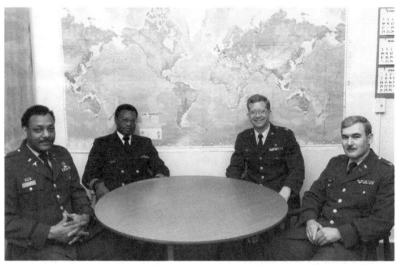

Figure 4-6. The first Armed Services Blood Program Blood Coordinating Committee (ABCC) established by Lieutenant Colonel Anthony Polk, Director of the Military Blood Program Office (MBPO) in 1985. From left to right: Lieutenant Colonel Anthony Polk, Lieutenant Commander Woody Woods, Captain Mike Ward, and Colonel James Spiker Jr. Courtesy of Colonel (Ret) Anthony Polk.

into various nonblood plans. For the first time, the joint strategic capability plan required a tab in all the medical annexes for blood. The US Transportation Command added a tab for blood shipments based on the time-phased force and deployment data list. The Armed Services Joint Medical Planning School in Norfolk added information on how wartime blood distribution was worked into its course of study. Unfortunately, since most logistics were handled by each individual service, planners and leaders had difficulty understanding how aspects of the blood program were integrated. Lieutenant Colonel Polk was tasked with providing a clear understanding of how the program was to work and briefing the Department of Defense medical executive council, which included the ASD(HA), the three surgeons general, the joint staff surgeon, combatant command surgeons, and others.

During his time in Vietnam, Lieutenant Colonel Polk had noted how well the Armed Services Medical Regulating System worked, and how well it was understood. Blood worked the same way, only in reverse. He visited the Armed Services Medical Regulating Service Office at Scott AFB to better understand their operations. The Armed Services Medical Regulating Service Office had established standardized Department of Defense names for the various elements of its system and placed them in Joint Publication 1-02, *Department of Defense Dictionary of*

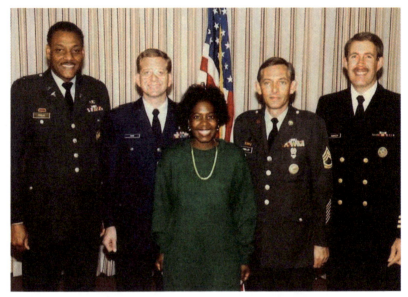

Figure 4-7. The first staff of the newly named Armed Services Blood Program Office (ASBPO) staff in 1987: (from left to right) Colonel Anthony Polk, Lieutenant Colonel Mike Ward, Ms. Ginger Rogers-Bass, Sergeant First Class Phil Winkler, and Commander Gerald Baker.

Military and Associated Terms.[6] Lieutenant Colonel Polk also liked the way the regulating system was laid out across CONUS and theater. This structure could be used for any of the unified commands.

Upon his return from Scott AFB, Lieutenant Colonel Polk drafted standard Department of Defense names for the military blood program, including the Armed Services Blood Program. He toyed with the idea of naming the program the "Armed Forces Blood Program" or "Defense Blood Program," but decided the Armed Services Blood Program was better understood and mirrored the Armed Services Medical Regulating Service Office. He also drafted a wartime blood distribution system, similar to the armed services medical regulating system. He presented the plans to the blood coordinating committee, which approved them. As a joint military activity, the Armed Services Blood Program (Figure 4-7) was similar to the existing Armed Services Medical Regulating Service in both terminology and structure. Afterward, Lieutenant Colonel Polk briefed the wartime blood distribution system to the medical executive council, with an understanding that most of the elements of the system were notional and had to be funded. The council members approved the concept and they instructed him to add the requirements into the Medical Readiness Strategic Plan.

The military blood community almost immediately began to use the new blood terminology. In 1987 the ASD(HA) released a worldwide message stating that the new terminology and blood distribution system would be used by all. Also, since policy at the time called for all peacetime efforts to support war, the new terminology migrated to the peacetime blood programs. Some pushback occurred, however, about officially changing the names of the respective service blood programs directors, such as the chief of the Air Force Blood Program. The compromise was to call the directors "service blood program officers" in a joint area, and retain their current titles within their services, according to Colonel (Retired) Anthony Polk's email dated March 2014.

A review of Army Medical Department doctrine resulted in the concept of Health Service Support, AirLand Battle, in 1986 (later changed to Health Service Support, AirLand Operations). The development of the revised doctrine continued into the 1990s. Medical Force 2000 changed how level III and IV units were organized. Deployable hospital equipment was changed from the Medical Unit Self-contained Transportable (MUST) configuration used during the Vietnam era to the new Deployable Medical Systems (DEPMEDS).[7] Changes would eventually come to the ABP as well.

As specified in the 1987 National Defense Authorization Act, the ASD(HA) directed that the initial Medical Readiness Strategic Plan be formulated.[5] The document was released in February 1988 and focused on correcting deficiencies in wartime medical readiness within 4 years. Unfortunately, over the next few years, the efforts of this plan were overcome by major events including the end of the Cold War and Operations Desert Shield and Desert Storm.

The implementation of a frozen blood program, which was an objective of MBP 2004, proved to be huge undertaking in terms of workload, technology, capital equipment, and resources for the ABP. The blood bank centers at Ft Hood and Ft Knox played an important role in the Army's frozen blood program. Lieutenant Colonel Stewart "Stu" Knodel (BBF class of '75–76) and Captain Jeff Schmidt (BBF class of '85–86) were the leads at the Ft Hood Blood Bank Center, and Lieutenant Colonel Ken Zielmanski (BBF class of '75–76) was the lead at the Camp Memorial Blood Center. Many in the ABP did not believe that frozen blood was a practical solution for the battlefield. Nonetheless, Colonel Platte led the ABP in procuring the latest ultra-low-temperature freezers and building facilities to house them. Large contracts with civilian blood centers were written to provide additional group O blood to freeze because most Army blood centers were challenged by their own transfusion requirements, according to Colonel (Retired) Richard Platte's email dated June 2014.

FOOD AND DRUG ADMINISTRATION LICENSING EXPANSION

In the latter part of the 1970s, FDA licensing was at the forefront of the ABP's goals, and by the end of the decade, several Army blood donor centers had already received FDA licenses. By the mid-1980s, the Army's FDA 611 license had continued to expand, and by the end of the decade a total of 22 Army facilities were on the license, according to Kathleen Elder's email dated February 2012.

Before additional locations were added to the license, the FDA added several new blood products to the Army's license, including platelet concentrate, added on January 15, 1982, and additive solutions, added in 1983. The additive solution blood collection systems use a second preservative solution for red cell storage, in addition to the primary anticoagulant, citrate-phosphate-dextrose (CPD) or citrate-phosphate-double dextrose (CP2D). These additives were specifically designed to further extend the shelf life of red blood cells. With the new technology, red blood cells could now be stored for 42 days, which was an increase from the 35-day shelf life of previous years. Captain Frank Rentas directed the Blood Bank Center–Ft Hood in 1996, when it became the first Army blood donor center to switch from CPDA-1 to AS-5 (Optisol; Terumo BCT Inc, Lakewood, CO), according to Colonel (Retired) Frank Rentas' telephone communication in June 2014. Two other 42-day additive solutions were available on the market at this time as well: AS-1 (Adsol; Fenwal Inc, Lake Zurich, IL) and AS-3 (Nutricel, Cutter Biological, Berkeley, CA).

By November 5, 1986, 22 Army facilities were on the Army's FDA 611 license. According to Kathleen Elder's email dated February 2012, these facilities included the following:

- Armed Services Blood Bank Center, Ft Ord, California
- Bassett US Army Community Hospital Blood Bank, Ft Wainwright, Alaska
- Bayne-Jones US Army Community Hospital Blood Bank, Ft Polk, Louisiana
- Brooke Army Medical Center, Ft Sam Houston, Texas
- Dwight David Eisenhower Army Medical Center, Ft Gordon, Georgia
- Evans US Army Community Hospital, Ft Carson, Colorado
- Fitzsimons Amy Medical Center, Denver, Colorado
- Frank R. Camp Memorial Blood Center, Ft Knox, Kentucky
- General Leonard Wood Army Community Hospital Blood Bank, Ft Leonard Wood, Missouri
- Irwin US Army Community Hospital Blood Bank, Ft Riley, Kansas
- Letterman Army Medical Center, Presidio of San Francisco, California

DEPARTMENT OF HEALTH & HUMAN SERVICES   Public Health Service

Food and Drug Administration
Bethesda MD 20892

DATE: Nov. 13, 1989

FROM: Donald Hill, Director, Division of Product
Certification, HFB-240 *Donald Hill*

SUBJECT: "Eight-Hour Hold"

TO: Blood and Plasma Inspectors, Center for
Biologics Evaluation and Research

THRU: Joel Solomon, Ph.D., Director, Division of Blood and
Blood Products, HFB-400

The Center for Biologics Evaluation and Research has approved recently an extension of the maximum room temperature hold period following collection of whole blood from six to eight hours prior to preparation of components.

Manufacturers of two blood collection systems submitted supplements to their New Drug Applications (NDAs) with data to support approval of the "eight-hour hold." These systems are the ADSOL^R solution system (anticoagulant CPD), manufactured by Fenwal Laboratories, Division of Baxter Healthcare Corporation and the Nutricel^R system (anticoagulant CP2D), manufactured by Cutter Biological, Division of Miles Inc. The systems have been generically termed as Additive Solution Systems because they utilize a second preservative solution for red blood cell storage in addition to the anticoagulant solution CPD or CP2D.

In both systems the Red Blood Cells may be separated from the plasma within eight hours after room temperature storage. Data submitted from platelets and Factor VIII studies of the plasma support that the plasma is suitable for the manufacture of Platelets, Fresh Frozen Plasma, Cryoprecipitated AHF, and Recovered Plasma.

Terumo Corporation, the manufacturer of the other marketed additive solution system, Optisol^R (anticoagulant CPD), is performing studies to prepare the submission of a supplemental application for the extension of the hold period to their NDA.

No manufacturer has received specific approval for the eight-hour hold for whole blood collected in CPDA-1 at this time. Baxter Healthcare Corp.'s supplemental application for the extension of the hold period to their CPDA-1 NDA is pending. Neither Cutter nor Terumo has submitted a request for the extension for CPDA-1.

Exhibit 4-1. Food and Drug Administration approval letter for "Eight-Hour Hold." November 13, 1989. Courtesy of the Army Blood Program Office.

- Madigan Army Medical Center, Tacoma, Washington
- Martin US Army Community Hospital Blood Bank, Ft Benning, Georgia
- Moncrieff US Army Community Hospital Blood Bank, Ft Jackson, South Carolina
- Noble US Army Community Hospital Blood Bank, Ft McClellan, Alabama
- Tripler Army Medical Center, Honolulu, Hawaii
- US Army Blood Bank Center, Ft Hood, Texas
- US Army Europe Blood Bank, Landstuhl, West Germany
- Walson US Army Community Hospital Blood Bank, Ft Dix, New Jersey
- Walter Reed Army Medical Center, Washington, DC
- William Beaumont Army Medical Center, El Paso, Texas
- Womack US Army Community Hospital Blood Bank, Ft Bragg, North Carolina

As the decade was ending, the ABP received more good news from the FDA. On November 13, 1989, the FDA allowed Army blood donor centers to separate red blood cells from plasma within 8 hours at room temperature storage (Exhibit 4-1). The announcement, released by an FDA memorandum titled "Eight-Hour Hold," meant that red blood cells could be separated from the plasma within 8 hours after room temperature storage if Fenwal's Adsol collection system (Fenwal Inc, Lake Zurich, IL) or Nutricel system (Cutter Biological, Division of Miles Laboratories, Emeryville, CA) were used, thus allowing Army blood donor centers an extra 2 hours to centrifuge donor units and place the plasma components into the freezer.[8] This was very helpful because most of the blood collections in the Army were through mobile blood drives, requiring the blood to be refrigerated before transport to the processing center; now refrigeration was no longer required during the 8-hour window.

INFECTIOUS DISEASE TESTING ADVANCES PROGRAM
Hepatitis

Before the 1980s, advances in infectious disease testing were just beginning within the civilian blood industry and the ABP. Tests for syphilis and hepatitis B were already implemented, but it was not until the mid-1980s that additional testing was added: two tests for screening indirect evidence of non-A and non-B hepatitis—the hepatitis B core antibody (1986) and the serum alanine aminotransferase liver test, more commonly known as ALT (1987)—were implemented across the United States.

Acquired Immune Deficiency Syndrome

Unusual cases of opportunistic diseases began to appear among homosexual men in 1981. In caring for these patients, doctors also discovered that the patients' immune systems were compromised. The condition soon began appearing in hemophiliac patients,[9] leading clinicians and scientists to believe that the condition could be transmitted through blood transfusions. This condition became known as acquired immune deficiency syndrome (AIDS). Dr. Robert Gallo published an article about the isolation of the retrovirus in 1983, originally called human T-cell lymphotropic virus III (HTLV-III), believed to be the cause of AIDS,[10] and later developed a blood test that provided the means to screen for the virus. This was the first time such a test could be performed. The virus was subsequently renamed the human immunodeficiency virus (HIV). In 1985, the FDA approved the first commercial blood test to detect antibodies to HIV, the enzyme-linked immunosorbent assay (ELISA), which was quickly implemented across the United States. Shortly thereafter, the Pentagon announced it would begin testing all new military recruits for HIV infection and reject those who tested positive. It was not until late in 1987 that the FDA required HIV testing on all donated blood[11]; in the interim 3 years, the FDA only recommended the testing. The delayed requirement drew criticism across the country as the number of AIDS cases increased.

During the next several years, Colonel Spiker (now at OTSG) and Lieutenant Colonel Gerald Jacobs, who served as the HSC laboratory and blood bank consultant from 1985 to 1988, were extremely busy. Together they had to ensure the safety of the current blood supply; ensure an HIV-negative donor base; develop a plan to test all active duty, National Guard, and Reserve soldiers; and establish the Army's biannual HIV testing program. Lieutenant Colonel Jacobs established a spreadsheet file to track HIV look-back cases in HSC, which was the precursor to many years of organizing and maintaining HIV look-back cases for the ABP. Eventually, new systems were created to manage the caseload, but at that point, Jacobs' spreadsheet was the only system in place.

Increased scrutiny by the FDA and new infectious disease testing were making blood banking increasingly more safe, but also more complicated. It soon became clear that a system of data automation was needed. The main drivers for an automated system were HIV look-back investigations. In 1986 Lieutenant Colonel John Bell, Army Medical Department Center & School, made a bold move to centrally purchase a blood bank computer system for the HSC. This system, considered to be one of the best for blood banks, was owned by a company called Western Star, according to Lieutenant Colonel (Retired) Robert Usry's email dated March 2014. However, the ASD(HA) discouraged the services from purchasing a commercial off-the-shelf system, according to Colonel (Retired) Jim Spiker's email dated March 2014. Efforts to purchase Western Star as an enterprise solution for the blood program were halted, and in 1987 the Armed Services Blood Program Office (ASBPO) formed a task force of blood bank officers from each service to begin building the Defense Blood Management Information System (DBMIS). However, the lack of computerization in those early years and the huge delay in implementing the system had a big impact on the ABP.

When Colonel Platte replaced Lieutenant Colonel Jacobs as the HSC clinical laboratory and blood bank consultant in October 1988, nearly 300 HIV look-back cases were being monitored. Most of the monitoring was performed manually in military treatment facilities with central coordination at the HSC. Colonel Platte convinced the HSC's commanding general to increase the ABP's efforts and resources to build a more robust HIV look-back computer program. By early 1989, the caseload had increased exponentially and HSC became inundated with cases of posttransfusion HIV infections. Although the DBMIS was still in development, it was not until 1994, when the Defense Blood Standard System (DBSS) (Figure 4-8) was introduced, that another information management system became available for HIV look-back investigations. Therefore, Colonel Platte intensified the HIV look-back program and hired Gloria Ochoa as the ABP's first look-back coordinator.

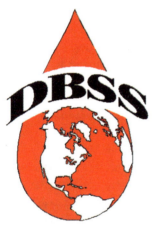

Figure 4-8. The Defense Blood Standard System (DBSS) logo/brand. Courtesy of the Armed Services Blood Program Office.

Colonel Platte developed a prototype HIV look-back computer program for central management of the HSC look-back cases by June 1990, yet the cases continued to mount. In February 1991 Colonel Platte made an urgent request to the Health Care Systems Support Agency (a field operating agency under HSC) to redesign, reprogram, and implement an automated database to serve the growing needs of the HSC and the Army Medical Department for HIV look-back investigations. Just as Colonel Platte departed for his next assignment in May 1993, the effort began to take shape.

The HIV look-back program uncovered several cases of posttransfusion HIV infections. Meanwhile, a new screening test for the detection of antibodies to another retrovirus, human T-cell lymphotropic virus I, or HTLV-I, was licensed and implemented across the United States. A February 28, 1989, ABP memorandum directed ABP blood donor centers to commence testing for HTLV-I no later than April 1, 1989.[12,13]

Although the decade brought great improvements and advancements in infectious disease testing, there was still a long road ahead to perfect the processes and management of the HIV look-back cases. In the early part of the 1990s, the HIV look-back program underwent several changes that helped the ABP regain control of the caseload.

SUMMARY

The 1980s saw a commitment to quality and a move toward improved joint medical operations. The Army Blood Program faced challenges in the AIDS epidemic and new military operations, but dedicated leaders continued pushing the program to become even better.

REFERENCES

1. US Department of the Army. *Military Blood Program Office*. Washington, DC: DA; 1980. Army Regulation 10-64.
2. US Department of Defense. *Military Blood Program*. Washington, DC: DoD; 1972. DoD Directive 6480.5.
3. US Department of the Army. *Relocation of the Armed Services Blood Bank Center (ASBBC) Fort Ord, CA, to Fort Lewis, WA*. Fort Sam Houston, TX: DA, Health Services Command. Staffing packet, April 23, 1993.
4. US Department of Defense. *Request for Blood Program Analysis*. Washington, DC: Military Field Medical Systems Standardization Steering Group. Letter, October 21, 1983.
5. US Department of Defense. *Medical Readiness Strategic Plan 1995–2001*. https://archive.org/details/MedicalReadinessStrategicPlan19952001. 1995. Accessed March 19, 2017.
6. US Department of Defense. *Department of Defense Dictionary of Military and Associated Terms*. Washington, DC: Department of Defense; 2017. Joint Publication 1-02. http://www.dtic.mil/doctrine/new_pubs/dictionary.pdf. Accessed April 26, 2017.
7. Ginn RVN. *The History of the US Army Medical Service Corps*. Washington, DC: DA, Office of The Surgeon General and Center of Military History; 1997.
8. Food and Drug Administration. *Eight-Hour Hold*. Bethesda, MD: Department of Health and Human Services. Memorandum, November 13, 1989.
9. Centers for Disease Control and Prevention. *Pneumocystic carinni* among persons with hemophilia A. *MMWR Morb Mortal Wkly Rep*. 1982;31:365–367.
10. Gallo RC, Sarin PS, Gelman EP, et al. Isolation of human T-cell leukemia virus in acquired deficiency syndrome (AIDS). *Science*. 1983;220:865–867.

11. US Food and Drug Administration. HIV/AIDS historical time line, 1981–1990. http://www.fda.gov/forpatients/illness/hivaids/history/ucm151074.htm. Updated August 8, 2014. Accessed April 27, 2017.
12. Office of The Surgeon General. *Implementation of Testing Blood Donations for HTLV-1*. Falls Church, VA: Department of the Army. Memorandum, February 28, 1989.
13. Armed Services Blood Program Office. *Guidelines for Testing Donated Blood for Antibodies to HTLV-1*. Falls Church, VA: Department of Defense. Memorandum, January 19, 1989.

ARMY REGULATION }
No. 10-64

AR 10-64

HEADQUARTERS
DEPARTMENT OF THE ARMY
WASHINGTON, DC, *15 May 1980*

ORGANIZATION AND FUNCTIONS
MILITARY BLOOD PROGRAM OFFICE
Effective 15 June 1980

This regulation implements DOD Directive 6480.5 and sets forth the mission and functions within the Department of the Army of the Military Blood Program Office. Local supplementation of this regulation is prohibited, except upon approval of The Surgeon General.

Interim changes to this regulation are not official unless they are authenticated by The Adjutant General. Users will destroy interim changes on their expiration dates unless sooner superseded or rescinded.

	Paragraph
Purpose	1
Applicability	2
Mission	3
Functions	4
Command and staff relationships	5
Other relationships	6

1. Purpose. This regulation sets forth the mission and principal functions of the Military Blood Program Office (MBPO).

2. Applicability. This regulation applies to all elements of the Active Army, Army National Guard, and US Army Reserve.

3. Mission. The mission of the MBPO is to coordinate the DOD Military Blood Program.

4. Functions. The principal functions of the MBPO are as follows:

  a. Monitor the implementation of the DOD Military Blood Program.

  b. Maintain and issue plans to coordinate the collection, processing, distribution, and management of blood and blood components of the Military Departments.

  c. Coordinate plans, policies, and procedures with the Military Departments and the unified and specified commands.

  d. Coordinate plans and actions which have military operational impact with the joint Chiefs of Staff.

  e. Prescribe information requirements as needed to ensure an effective blood program.

  f. Advise the Defense Logistics Agency (DLA) on the following matters:

    (1) Procurement of whole blood and blood components.

    (2) Mobilization and industrial mobilization needs for natural and synthetic plasma expanders.

  g. Develop, recommend, and monitor coordinated policies to—

    (1) Collect, procure, process, store, issue, and manage whole blood.

    (2) Determine acceptability, issue, and use of blood components and synthetic or other nonhuman plasma volume expanders.

  h. Request emergency and mobilization military needs for whole blood from the Military Departments and unified and specified commands; determine net DOD requirements.

  i. Approve guides on blood banking which will be used as minimum standards by the Military Departments.

Attachment 4-1.

AR 10-64

j. Coordinate with the Defense Medical Materiel Board on essential characteristics of blood bank equipment and reagents.

k. Act on oversea requests from theater commanders for whole blood and blood components and on CONUS requests which exceed the resources of the Military Departments.

l. When authorized by the Assistant Secretary of Defense (Health Affairs) (ASD(HA)), request that DLA use standby contracts to procure blood from civilian sources. This will occur when Military Department needs exceed internal blood collections and processing.

m. Coordinate research and development needs of the DOD Military Blood Program. Submit these needs through ASD(HA) to the Director of Defense Research and Engineering (DDRE).

n. Coordinate technical aspects of blood research programs when requested by DDRE.

5. Command and staff relationships. *a.* The MBPO is a Joint Service element under the operational control of The Surgeon General (TSG), HQDA.

b. The Director of the MBPO is appointed by the Surgeons General of the Army, Navy, and Air Force. This appointment must have the concurrence of the ASD(HA). Other members of the MBPO will be designated deputy directors. They will represent their respective Military Department and have direct access to their Surgeon General.

c. The ASD(HA) provides policy guidance on the DOD Military Blood Program, and coordinates it with the Federal Emergency Management Agency.

6. Other relationships. *a.* The Secretary of the Army, in support of the DOD Military Blood Program, will—

(1) Maintain operational control of the MBPO.

(2) Provide administrative support for the internal administration and operation of the MBPO.

(3) Program, budget, and finance all MBPO operating costs. This does not include the pay, allowances, and PCS travel of military members and assigned staff. These funds are provided by the respective Military Departments.

(4) Fund for blood procurement from civilian sources to include the cost of transportation to the Armed Services Whole Blood Processing Laboratory. This procurement may be made when military needs exceed supply. A Military Department may obtain blood and blood components by local purchase in any emergency where time or other considerations make such purchase desirable.

b. The Director, MBPO will provide direct liaison with other Government and civilian agencies on matters involving blood and related items.

2

Attachment 4-1. Continued

AR 10-64

> The proponent agency of this regulation is the Office of The Surgeon General. Users are invited to send comments and suggested improvements on DA Form 2028 (Recommended Changes to Publications and Blank Forms) direct to HQDA (DASG-PSC), WASH DC 20310.

By Order of the Secretary of the Army:

E. C. MEYER
General, United States Army
Chief of Staff

Official:
J. C. PENNINGTON
Major General, United States Army
The Adjutant General

DISTRIBUTION:

To be distributed in accordance with DA Form 12-9A, requirements for AR, Organization and Functions.
    Active Army—B
    USAR & ARNG—D

Attachment 4-1. Continued

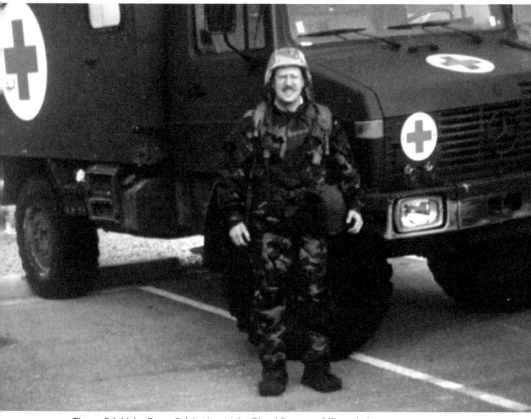

Figure 5-1. Major Bruce Sylvia, Area Joint Blood Program Officer, during Operations Desert Shield and Desert Storm. Courtesy of the Armed Services Blood Program Office.

CHAPTER FIVE

Testing Advances and Quality Assurance: 1990s

The new decade brought the start of military struggles throughout the Middle East. In the midst of Operations Desert Shield and Desert Storm, the Army Blood Program (ABP) moved forward with post–Cold War review and modernization, Food and Drug Administration (FDA) licensing, and infectious disease testing advancements. It also introduced new quality assurance measures to provide greater assurance that blood collected was safe to be shipped overseas and transfused worldwide.

FACILITY STATUS AND PROGRAM LEADERSHIP IN THE EARLY 1990s

Health Services Command (HSC) had 21 licensed facilities and 38 registered facilities by November 1992 (Attachment 5-1). The Walson US Army Community Hospital Blood Bank (Ft Dix) was removed from the Army FDA 611 license in 1992 when it was transferred to the Air Force (McGuire Air Force Base) and renamed Walson Air Force Hospital at the recommendation of the BRAC (Base Realignment and Closure) Commission. On April 30, 2001, Walson Hospital closed its doors as the Air Force vacated the building, according to Kathleen Elder's email dated January 2012.

Lieutenant Colonel Richard Brown (US Army Blood Bank Fellowship [BBF] class of '80–81) moved to the Office of The Surgeon General (OTSG) to replace Major Mike Stanton in 1991. After Colonel Jim Spiker retired, Major Stanton was tasked to cover the Blood Program Office at OTSG. He reported to Colonel Robert Pick, who had replaced Colonel Spiker as OTSG laboratory consultant. Lieutenant Colonel Brown oversaw policies while Colonel Richard Platte remained in charge of blood program operations until his departure from

HSC in May 1993, according to Colonel (Retired) Platte's email dated November 2011. Colonel Spiker realized early that the split between policy and operations would eventually change, and he brought Major Stanton into the operations and planning side of OTSG to begin the transition, according to Colonel (Retired) Richard Brown's email dated June 2014.

OPERATIONS DESERT SHIELD AND DESERT STORM

The Middle East has a long history of turmoil ranging from ethnic, tribal, religious, and geographic conflict to oil disputes. Beginning in July 1990, Iraq and Kuwait disagreed over oil consumption and pumping. One month later approximately 100,000 Iraqi troops moved into Kuwait followed by a United Nations demand for Iraq's withdrawal. At this point, it seemed that US involvement in the region was inevitable, so the ABP began to plan ahead.

Operation Desert Shield began when President George H.W. Bush ordered 200,000 US forces to the Persian Gulf region in early August. The deployment of troops began with the 2,300 soldiers from the 82nd Airborne Division. They deployed with a contingency shipment of O-negative red blood cells that HSC blood donor centers rushed to supplement. Later in August, the 24th Mechanized Infantry Division from Ft Stewart, Georgia, arrived in Saudi Arabia.[1]

The European Command (EUCOM) joint blood program officer, Major G. Michael Fitzpatrick (BBF class of '80–81), began working with the Armed Services Blood Program Office (ASBPO) on the blood support plan and requirements because the US Central Command (CENTCOM) did not have a blood bank officer on staff. In August, XVIII Airborne Corps medical units (44th Medical Brigade) deployed to the region. The 47th Field Hospital, the 28th Combat Support Hospital, and the 5th Mobile Army Surgical Hospital were under the command and control of the 44th Medical Brigade. Lieutenant Colonel Wilbur Malloy (BBF class of '76–77) deployed to Saudi Arabia to establish a frozen blood depot at Al Jubail. The biggest theater challenge for the frozen blood program was maintaining sufficient quantities of freezers and deglycerolization bowls, according to Lieutenant Colonel Wilbur Malloy's email dated April 2012.

It soon became clear that the ABP would play a critical role in the conflict. Colonel Richard Platte sent a message to all HSC blood donor centers to dust off their mobilization plans. Shortly thereafter, as the situation in theater deteriorated and conflict became likely, Colonel Platte ordered HSC medical centers and selected medical activities' blood donor centers to activate their plans.

In September, the 655th Medical Company (Blood Bank) in Germany deployed a team consisting of one officer (Captain Bob Borowski) and 17 enlisted soldiers. It took some time for all of the team's equipment to arrive in theater. When the team was operational it was collocated with the frozen blood depot in Al Jubail. The 335th Medical Company deployed from Germany to augment the 655th.[2]

To help with the heavy workload, two Army mobilization augmentees were assigned to assist Colonel Platte with the mobilization plans. Retired Lieutenant Colonel John Bell (BBF class of '73–74), a seasoned blood banker, was also brought in as a retiree recall. Colonel Platte saw that the interim OTSG blood program officer, Major Mike Stanton, was also becoming overextended. He convinced Brigadier General James Peake to recall retired Colonel Jim Spiker to active duty to work in the OTSG blood office, according to Colonel (Retired) Richard Platte's email dated November 2011. Colonel Spiker was brought back on active duty in November 1990, as a retiree recall, and remained activated until May 31, 1991, after all Operation Desert Storm after-action reviews were completed.

Later in September, the 135th Medical Company (blood bank) deployed its NC detachment (blood distribution) from Ft Bragg, North Carolina, to Dhahran, Saudi Arabia. Throughout the force buildup, four additional Army reserve blood supply units deployed to Southwest Asia: the 379th Blood Bank Company from Folsom, Pennsylvania; the 448th NA detachment (blood processing) from Des Moines, Iowa; the 387th NC detachment (blood distribution) from Brooklyn, New York; and the 605th NC detachment (blood distribution) from Des Moines, Iowa.[2] Also, the remaining team of the 655th Medical Company back in Germany prepared to begin freezing blood for EUCOM.

As Operation Desert Shield continued, the blood requirements placed on HSC outstripped the current capabilities to collect at the licensed establishments. Colonel Platte ordered the activation of an additional 11 contingency blood donor centers, at locations including Ft Belvoir, Virginia; Ft Eustis, Virginia; Ft Meade, Maryland; West Point, New York; and Ft Lee, Virginia. Most of these sites outsourced their blood donor testing to FDA-licensed civilian testing facilities, and Colonel Platte consolidated other East Coast testing to the Camp Memorial Blood Center at Ft Knox. One of the biggest challenges encountered at this phase was that mobilization equipment and supplies prepositioned at small nondonor center medical activities were often obsolete or inadequate. The ABP had to perform many emergency procurement actions to bring these centers up to standards.

Early in the mobilization, major flaws were found with the HSC mobilization plan for blood donor centers, despite annual exercises that had worked well. The plan was based on some invalid assumptions, including expectations that Forces Command installations would collect blood and troops would donate before deployment. Colonel Platte encountered some refusal from commanders to allow troops to donate blood while focusing on predeployment training and other preparations, and concerns arose that predeployment vaccinations might prevent troops from donating. This was especially true at Ft Hood, where the ABP had a major blood donor center. Colonel Platte therefore initiated the difficult task of moving the whole blood collection operation from Ft Hood to Ft Sill to reduce the percentage of potential donors disqualified in the screening process. Additionally, Tripler Army Medical Center was cleaved from operational control under HSC and transferred to US Army Western Command (the Army component of the Pacific Command, which later evolved into US Army Pacific) during Operation Desert Shield, removing one licensed facility from those available to support the Army in meeting its portion of CENTCOM blood requirements. The mobilization plan for blood donor centers had to be scrapped and a new plan created as the operation continued to escalate, according to Colonel (Retired) Richard Platte's email dated June 2014.

Blood collections at many licensed blood centers were severely curtailed by readiness planning. To make up for the drop in blood collections, the ABP had to rely heavily on several US Army Training and Doctrine Command (TRADOC) installations such as Ft Leonard Wood, Ft Sill, and, most notably, Ft Knox. With collections taking place throughout the country, the bulk of the collections still came from the Camp Memorial Blood Center, under the direction of Lieutenant Colonel Ken Zielmanski. Ft Knox was a large training base with an established blood center, whose staff proved capable of handling the increased workload.

As an additional measure, ASBPO discussed with Colonel Platte a plan for the Blood Bank Center at Ft Hood to rejuvenate and freeze blood to help meet some of the projected requirements. The biggest challenge, however, was the availability of sufficient quantities of PIPA (pyruvate, inosine, phosphate, and adenine) solution. During storage, frozen red cells begin to lose ATP (adenosine triphosphate) and 2,3-diphosphoglycerate, vital biochemicals needed for cell metabolism and the ability to transport oxygen. PIPA was a rejuvenation solution that would bring these biochemical levels up during the thawing and deglycerolization process. Significant quantities of this solution did not exist because manufacturing capacity was not available to process large quantities of frozen red cells in a relatively short period of time such as wartime. A final obstacle was the discontinuation of civilian blood collection on military installations. Although the ASBPO favored allowing these collections to continue, Colonel Platte believed civilian collections decreased the Army's ability to meet collection requirements, so he suspended civilian blood agencies' access to Army posts, according to Colonel (Retired) Richard Platte's email dated November 2011.

In November 1990, to fill the vacancy in blood support when the 655th and the 335th medical companies deployed to theater, several reserve units were alerted for possible deployment to Germany: the 548th NA detachment (blood processing), Madison, Wisconsin; the 325th NB detachment (blood collecting) from Mesquite, Texas; the 1467th NC detachment (blood distribution) from Ft Allen, Puerto Rico; and the 324th NB detachment (blood collecting) from Chester, Pennsylvania.[2] On December 26, Major Bruce Sylvia (Figure 5-1) (BBF class of '84–85) arrived in theater to serve as the area joint blood program officer, under the CENTCOM Joint Blood Program Office of Major Springer, US Air Force, and Lieutenant Commander Fieldman, US Navy, according to Colonel (Retired) Bruce Sylvia's email dated November 2011.

On January 12, 1991, Congress agreed to allow the president to use force to end the Persian Gulf crisis. By this time, the Army Medical Department (AMEDD) had deployed 44 hospitals and six blood supply units to Southwest Asia. After several months of intense preparation, the ABP was poised to meet the blood requirements of Operation Desert Storm (Figure 5-2). The program moved a considerable amount of blood to the Armed Services Whole Blood Processing Laboratory–East before the commencement of the air campaign on January 17, 1991. By the time the active war began, a total of 30,000 units of red blood cells from the three services, EUCOM, PACOM, and civilian sources was available in theater.

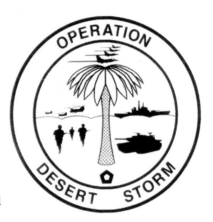

Figure 5-2. Logo of Operation Desert Storm. Courtesy of the Armed Services Blood Program Office.

In the months that followed, the blood pipeline began flowing well. When the ground invasion began on February 23, 1991, the ABP had provided most of the military blood collected to support the operation. During the 8 months of operations, the military collected and procured from civilian facilities approximately 105,000 units of red blood cells. This amount was derived from a planning factor of four units of packed red blood cells per wounded in action and nonbattle injury. The majority of blood was flown to CENTCOM and a smaller amount was flown to EUCOM using the Collins box, designed during the Vietnam War, as the shipping container. EUCOM's inventory was increased to support the wounded that would be evacuated out of theater.

In addition to frozen red blood cells, the 655th maintained liquid packed red blood cells and fresh frozen plasma. Blood products were provided to the Navy offshore, a field hospital in Bahrain, a forward deployed Marine medical

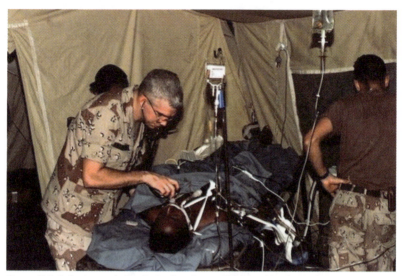

Figure 5-3. Patient care during Operations Desert Shield and Desert Storm. Courtesy of the Armed Services Blood Program Office.

unit, and other medical treatment facilities. During the actual assault, group O red blood cells were pushed forward. By the middle of February, more than 7,500 units of frozen red cells were in theater.[2] The 655th reported that from February 24 to 25, 235 frozen red cell units were deglycerolized, according to Lieutenant Colonel (Retired) Wilbur Malloy's email dated July 2014. Also, Navy personnel on the USNS *Mercy* deglycerolized 265 units. However, none of these units was transfused in part because of the limited shelf life (24 hours) of the unit postdeglycerolization.[3]

By the end of combat operations, deployed military hospitals had transfused approximately 2,000 units of red blood cells, 250 to injured US service members and the remainder to injured Iraqi civilians (Figure 5-3). Many Army hospitals deployed because the United States was expecting huge casualties once the conflict started. Although the ABP was prepared for the worst, the ground war lasted only 100 hours. The United States quickly overwhelmed Saddam Hussein and his army, and America suffered relatively few casualties. As blood expired at individual medical treatment facilities in theater, it was burned along with other medical waste. As hospitals began to close and redeploy, in-date blood products were shipped to other military hospitals that were still operational.

On February 28, 1991, a cessation of hostilities was declared. The terms of the ceasefire were negotiated in Safwan, Iraq, on March 1, 1991. Iraq accepted the terms on April 6, 1991, with an effective date of April 11, 1991.[1]

In an after-action review, several issues and concerns from operations within theater arose that the ABP would have to address in the coming years, according to Lieutenant Colonel (Retired) Wilbur Malloy's email dated July 2014:
- The Theater Army Medical Management Information System for medical logistics did not work. As a result, blood supply units had to use Microsoft Excel spreadsheets, dot matrix printers, and computers to manage the inventory and distribution.
- There was a high breakage rate with the fresh frozen plasma.
- The bar codes on military-collected units versus civilian-collected units were different, which made scanning difficult.
- No biomedical maintenance support for laboratory equipment was available. Blood supply units had to rely on host country support.
- Ice making capability was insufficient.
- The planning factors used were based on a European Cold War scenario. For the length and type of operation that Operation Desert Storm became, there was a huge available inventory for the amount of units actually transfused.
- Personnel were confused about the roles of the 30th Medical Brigade and 44th Medical Brigade in support of the blood depot.
- Approval to provide blood support to host nations was required (eg, the 655th provided a large amount of blood to a host nation hospital in support of an auto accident victim), but the actual approving authority was unclear.
- Transportation assets for delivery of blood products were limited, causing problems moving blood products from the air head to the depot and from the depot to forward medical units.

MANDATES OF THE BASE REALIGNMENT AND CLOSURE COMMISSION

The BRAC Act of 1991 recommended the closure of Ft Ord. With that directive, the Armed Services Blood Bank Center at Ft Ord (the first tri-service blood donor center) closed in September 1993. Its personnel were transferred to Madigan Army Medical Center to help build a new facility in the Pacific Northwest.[4] With the closure and personnel transfer, however, the Navy decided to withdraw from the original memorandum of understanding, so the new Armed Services Blood Bank Center at Ft Lewis consisted only of Army and Air Force personnel. Lieutenant Colonel Dave Miller (BBF class of '86–87) was the last director at Ft Ord, according to Colonel Steve Beardsley's email dated March 2011.

In 1992, the Army focused on reorganizing the AMEDD. In September, the new surgeon general, Lieutenant General Alcide LaNoue, presented a concept plan to Army headquarters that would realign the AMEDD. Among the outcomes was a single command structure for Army medicine, the US Army Medical Command (MEDCOM). In August 1993, the Army chief of staff, General Gordon Sullivan, approved the plan, and in October MEDCOM (Provisional) began a 1-year process of replacing the HSC. MEDCOM became fully operational in October 1994. Under this command, management and oversight of medical treatment facilities were consolidated. The surgeon general now wore two hats—the surgeon general's traditional role as senior medical advisor on the Army staff was combined with command authority over MEDCOM and its subordinate units.[5,6]

During this time of significant change, the ABP was decentralized and standard operating procedures were established by each individual blood bank. However, quality assurance positions at each blood bank were nonexistent. The FDA also started using 21 CFR Part 211,[7] in addition to Part 600,[8] making blood establishments operate more like pharmaceutical companies. The AMEDD was downsizing at the same time federal requirements on the blood program were increasing. Since there would not be enough personnel to match the requirements, Lieutenant Colonel Brown and the existing staff would have to learn many new responsibilities to effectively implement the program.

In May 1993, as HSC was deactivated and the new MEDCOM became fully operational, Colonel Platte departed San Antonio and became the executive officer for the Armed Forces Institute of Pathology in Washington, DC. He retired from the Army the following year, in December 1994. The same year Lieutenant Colonel Brown was directed to move the Army Blood Program Office (ABPO) to MEDCOM. The consolidation of OTSG and HSC established a single ABPO at MEDCOM with oversight of both policy and operations. Under Lieutenant Colonel Brown's leadership as director of the Army Blood Program, the Army's FDA license structure was reorganized. The surgeon general would be the responsible person on the Army's FDA blood establishment, and the director of the ABP would be the alternate responsible person.

A few years later, in 1996, Fitzsimons Army Medical Center began closure because of the BRAC Act of 1995. Major Donna Whittaker closed the facility's blood program, according to Kathleen Elder's email dated March 2012. After this closure, there were 19 611-licensed facilities in the Army (Exhibit 5-1).

DEPARTMENT OF HEALTH AND HUMAN SERVICES
WASHINGTON, D.C.

ESTABLISHMENT LICENSE
FOR THE MANUFACTURE OF BIOLOGICAL PRODUCTS

This is to certify that Establishment License No. _____611_____ is hereby issued to _____Department of the Army_____, the manufacturer, located at _____Washington, DC_____, through the establishment identified as _____Department of the Army_____ located at _____Washington, DC_____ with __19__ locations which follow,

Bassett U.S Army Community Hospital Blood Bank, Fort Wainwright, Alaska
Bayne-Jones U S Army Community Hospital Blood Bank, Fort Polk, Louisiana
Brooke Army Medical Center, Fort Sam Houston, Texas
Dwight David Eisenhower Army Medical Center, Fort Gordon, Georgia
Evans Army Community Hospital, Fort Carson, Colorado
Frank R Camp Memorial Blood Center, Fort Knox, Kentucky
General Leonard Wood U S Army Community Hospital Blood Bank,
  Fort Leonard Wood Missouri
Irwin U S Army Community Hospital Blood Bank, Fort Riley, Kansas
Armed Services Blood Bank Center, Tacoma, Washington
Martin U S Army Community Hospital Blood Bank, Fort Benning, Georgia
Moncrief U S Army Community Hospital Blood Bank Fort Jackson, South Carolina
Tripler Army Medical Center, Honolulu, Hawaii
U S Army Blood Bank Center Fort Hood, Texas
USA MEDDAC, West Point, New York
USAREUR Blood Donor Center, Landstuhl, West Germany
USFK Blood Center, Seoul, Korea
Walter Reed Army Medical Center Washington, DC
William Beaumont Army Medical Center, El Paso, Texas
Womack Army Medical Center Fort Bragg, North Carolina

pursuant to Section 351 of the Public Health Service Act, approved July 1, 1944 (58 Stat. 702, 42 U.S.C. 262), as amended, and the regulations thereunder. The license authorizes the manufacturer to maintain an establishment for the propagation or manufacture and preparation for sale, barter, or exchange in the District of Columbia, or for sending, carrying, or bringing for sale, barter, or exchange from any State or possession into any other State or possession or into any foreign country, or from any foreign country into any State or possession, any virus, therapeutic serum, toxin, antitoxin, vaccine, blood, blood component or derivative, allergenic product, or analogous product, or arsphenamine or its derivatives, for which the manufacturer holds an unsuspended and unrevoked product license issued by the Secretary of Health and Human Services pursuant to said Act and regulations.

Date October 10, 1996

Director, Center for Biologics
Evaluation and Research
Food and Drug Administration

Exhibit 5-1. Food and Drug Administration Establishment License 611. October 10, 1996. Courtesy of the Army Blood Program Office.

POST–COLD WAR REVIEW

In September 1992, ASBPO convened a conference panel with representation from all three services to conduct a formal review of the entire peacetime, contingency, and wartime program. The panel provided 28 recommendations that eventually were incorporated into the Medical Readiness Strategic Plan (MRSP) 2001. One recommendation was to review the procedures for providing random group O Rh-positive and group O Rh-negative at echelon two in relation to the increasing roles of women on the battlefield. Another recommendation was to reexamine the accuracy of blood types on identification cards and tags.[9]

In 1993 the AMEDD began a new modernization effort to transform its deployable units. With force reductions and lessons learned from Operations Desert Shield and Desert Storm, the AMEDD saw a need for units to be farther forward on the battlefield, more flexible, and able to conduct split-based operations. The new effort was known as the medical reengineering initiative and it continued well into the next decade.

Many changes had occurred in the post–Cold War period, including a booming economy and the rapid development and expansion of information technology, especially the internet. With the collapse of the Soviet Union and the threat of communism dramatically reduced, the nation's defense planning guidance also changed. No longer would America plan to contain the Soviet Union, but rather it would focus more on regional threats. In 1994, the ASD(HA) reexamined the original MRSP released in 1988. A new document, MRSP 2001, placed an emphasis on planning and execution of medical readiness objectives through 2001 and beyond. The plan was divided into nine initial functional areas. The ASBP was the lead on the following five action plans:

1. **ASBP**. The 1992 ASBP update conference panel had agreed that a "centralized blood program management system must exist to ensure efficient use of blood resources and meet FDA requirements."[9]
2. **Joint blood doctrine**. Blood program doctrine must meet the evolving joint and combined doctrine. The joint blood distribution system was "published in Joint Pub 4-02 Doctrine for Health Service Support in Joint Operations. Technical procedures were included in Joint Pub 4-02.1 Health Service Support Logistics in Joint Operations. Additionally, the proper usage and distribution of blood products was inserted into DEPMEDS policies."[9]
3. **Peacetime operations**. The services' blood programs had to change business practices to meet new FDA quality assurance guidelines and requirements under the Clinical Laboratory Improvement Amendments of 1988. Also, deglycerolized frozen red cells must be included in major

hospital inventories to be used as an additional blood product for treating patients. Additionally, all research and development efforts must continue.
4. **Wartime operations.** Using lessons learned from Operations Desert Shield, Desert Storm, and Restore Hope, the ASBP must ensure efficiencies and continued improvements throughout the programs.
5. **Research and development.** The services must continue specified research and development initiatives, including extended shelf-life red blood cells, extended shelf life platelets, technology to collect platelets in a field environment, extended shelf life of deglycerolized red blood cells, and blood substitutes as a way to reduce the risks of infectious diseases.

The Army and Navy were the service leads on the action plan for frozen blood. The operation plan noted that frozen blood would be used to mitigate any shortfalls in packed red blood cells. This supported one of the recommendations from the 1992 ASBP update conference and established prepositioned strategic locations within EUCOM, PACOM, and CENTCOM.[9]

The blood functional area in MRSP 2001 had 52 tasks, and almost all were completed or on schedule. Key goals that affected the ABP included the following[10]:
- establish an FDA-compliant quality assurance programs;
- license all DoD collection facilities with the FDA;
- update blood doctrine to meet combatant command requirements (Joint Publication 4-02.1[11]);
- establish field collection capabilities;
- complete frozen blood fielding in the combatant commands; and
- develop and field Defense Blood Standard System (DBSS).

While serving as the deputy director for operations at ASBPO, Lieutenant Colonel Noel Webster was responsible for drafting and staffing a new Health Affairs policy for using identification cards and tags for emergency transfusions. He included new information gained from the 1992 ASBP update conference. Specifically, the policy stated that at echelon two, the services will provide Rh negative red cells to Rh negative males and females based on the blood type on their identification cards and tags. Since higher echelons of care had capabilities to type and cross match, providers were to give group-specific Rh negative red cells for Rh negative males and females. The policy also directed that if a shortage of Rh negative blood occurred, priority should be given to Rh negative females as a means to reduce Rh sensitization in women of child-bearing years, according to Colonel (Retired) Steve Beardsley's email dated February 2014.

The practice of having a soldier's blood type on his or her identification card can be traced to World War II. It enabled rapid blood type determination during an emergency if an individual required a transfusion or was needed as a donor. To prevent transfusion reactions from blood typing errors, cross matching the blood before transfusion was still required, except in extreme emergencies.[12] Kendrick noted that during World War II, blood typing errors on identification tags ranged between 5% and 25%.[13] In 1988, Colonel Polk participated in a group that studied blood typing errors on identification cards and tags; the group found an error rate of approximately 11%.[14] As a result of the continuing problem of inaccurate blood typing, the new ASD(HA) policy directed the services to review their procedures for validating blood types and ensure that the blood type on a soldier's identification card and tag matched a laboratory result in his or her medical record.[15]

On January 7, 1998, a Health Affairs health operations policy letter to the surgeons general requested the services to consider consolidating blood donor center functions and quality assurance programs. During an ASBPO Blood Coordinating Committee meeting in June of the same year, service blood program leaders developed operational recommendations, five of which were specific to the Army:
1. Close the Ft Riley donor center.
2. Evaluate moving the Camp Memorial Blood Center to Ft Jackson due to a significant change in its donor population.
3. Keep the WRAMC donor center open until the establishment of an Armed Services Blood Bank Center in the national capitol area.
4. Consolidate blood donor testing at Ft Knox, Ft Hood, and Ft Lewis.
5. Make the donor center at Landstuhl, Germany, the EUCOM blood donor center.

The committee also discussed the establishment of a consolidated donor center in San Antonio at Lackland AFB with Air Force and Navy staff. At the time, the Army did not see any benefits to merging into this group, but agreed to reexamine the possibility in the future.[16]

In August 1998, the ASD(HA) released MRSP 1998–2004, which was a review and update to MRSP 2001. Thirty specific tasks were identified for the ASBP, many of which were the same as in the previous plan. However, some new tasks emerged, including the following:
- develop and deploy a year 2000 (Y2K) compliant DBSS on the Windows NT operating system;
- establish joint-consolidated blood centers for the most efficient manufacturing, testing, and operations;

- assess the possibility of maximizing plasma recovery from whole blood in order to support contract agreements with American Red Cross to provide plasma in return for SD plasma (best for virus deactivation);
- obtain and deploy an automated blood product labeling system (for on-demand printing) for DBSS;
- provide Theater-DBSS and joint total asset visibility;
- determine requirement and planning factors in a nuclear, biological, and chemical environment;
- develop sterilization and rapid infectious disease detection techniques; and
- develop a process for automated field production of water for processes such as blood product washing and reconstitution.[10]

NEW TESTING AND QUALITY ASSURANCE REQUIREMENTS

In 1990 the blood industry implemented a new antibody test, for hepatitis C (the agent believed to be the main source of non-A, non-B hepatitis), just 2 years after the virus was identified. The first generation (version 1.0) assay was not perfect; it had low sensitivity and a relatively high false positive rate. It took another 2 years before the assay was improved (version 2.0), significantly reducing the virus from the blood supply.[17]

The FDA held a workshop in Silver Spring, Maryland, to announce its draft guidelines for quality assurance in blood establishments in 1991. This draft, which was eventually issued in a final format in 1995,[18] caused an upheaval in the US blood industry and was not widely accepted. The meeting was confrontational, but it gave the industry a clear picture of where it was heading. Previously, the American Association of Blood Banks (known today as the AABB) provided guidance for the industry. The FDA deferred to the AABB's *Standards for Blood Banks and Transfusion Services* and, in most instances, blood was considered a service to be delivered to the patient under the professional oversight of pathologists. With the new draft guideline, the FDA declared it would begin to govern the blood industry and AABB would be subordinate to the FDA. The FDA indicated it would also invoke 21 CFR Part 211 documents, which contain the current good manufacturing practices requirements for finished pharmaceuticals,[7] in addition to 21 CFR Part 600, which deals with biological products.[8] The blood products manufactured within the US blood industry could now be regulated as biological products as well as drugs. This major change quickly had a significant impact on blood donor centers and transfusion services.

In September 1992, the ABP directed all blood donor centers and transfusion services to establish a quality improvement program based on the FDA's draft guidelines for quality assurance.[19] A key requirement was the creation of a dedicated quality improvement unit or individual with direct reporting authority. Each facility was instructed to implement the program according to specific local requirements. Blood donor centers and transfusion services were also given the authority to shut down operations if they determined that critical processes were no longer in control (not following the manufacturer's directions and standard operating procedures).

The regulatory oversight of the blood industry rapidly expanded, in part because of the HIV epidemic. Under the Federal Food, Drug, and Cosmetic Act, the FDA is empowered to enforce federal regulations that pertain to the blood industry, including the right to conduct unannounced inspections of all blood facilities regardless of licensure status.[20] For military donor centers overseas, the FDA coordinated with the ABPO for available dates and installation access. Because of these inspections, the ABPO developed a standardized checklist to help facilities during and after an inspection.[21] On July 11, 1995 (several years after draft guidance was initially discussed), the FDA published *Guidelines for Quality Assurance in Blood Establishments*.[18] The purpose of these guidelines was to assist manufacturers of blood and blood components, including blood banks, transfusion services, and plasmapheresis centers, in developing a quality assurance program to be consistent with recognized principles of quality assurance and current good manufacturing practices. Because blood and blood components are drugs under the Food, Drug, and Cosmetic Act, the current good manufacturing practices regulations in 21 CFR Parts 210 and 211 are applicable. In addition, the FDA issued regulations for blood and blood components in 21 CFR Part 606 intended to be used in conjunction with the applicable federal standards in 21 CFR Parts 600 through 680 and Parts 210 and 211, according to Colonel (Retired) Richard Brown in his email dated February 2012.

The ABP issued several revised recommendations in 1992 to reduce HIV transmission by transfusion.[22] Among the recommendations were the following:

- Conduct a private and confidential health history interview with each prospective donor and ensure that the high-risk behavior questions are asked "verbatim" as established by the FDA.
- Establish and retain a confidential unit exclusion procedure to provide an additional means for individuals to self-exclude their donation when peer pressure may prevent them from self-exclusion during the donor interview process. Peer pressure was a concern especially during blood drives held for military units.
- Provide HIV educational material to each prospective donor.
- "Implement HIV-2 testing in accordance with the ASBPO/Health Affairs deadline."[22] HIV-2 is a different virus, but in the same family as the virus that caused the AIDS epidemic, now referred to as HIV-1.

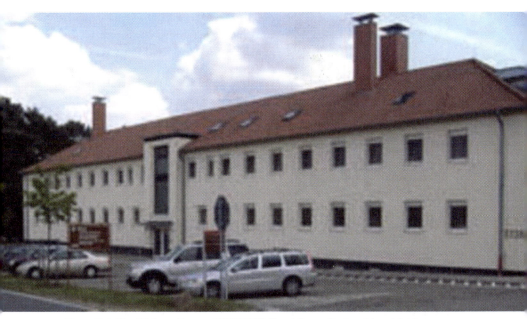

Figure 5-4. The US Army Europe (USAREUR) Blood Donor Center at Landstuhl, Germany, circa 2001. Courtesy of the Armed Services Blood Program Office.

The ABP also announced the FDA licensure of a supplemental anti-hepatitis C virus (HCV) test for repeat reactive donors in November 1993.[23] However, Army blood donor centers were not required to implement the test because it was still being evaluated by the FDA. Instead, centers were told to maintain the same testing algorithm and donor deferral criteria from the previous HCV testing policy. Repeat reactive donors were permanently deferred.

By the 1990s, the HIV look-back program caseload had been reduced and was starting to track other infectious diseases. Colonel Richard Brown hired John Ives to replace Gloria Ochoa as the HIV look-back coordinator in 1994. John Ives held this position until his retirement in 2002, when Sergeant Major (Retired) Anselmo "Papo" Martinez became the next coordinator.

On August 9, 1995, an ABP policy memorandum[24] announced that Army blood donor centers were no longer required to perform alanine aminotransferase liver testing on units of blood donated for transfusion purposes. A December 13, 1995, ABP memorandum[25] outlined the testing algorithms and donor deferral management for HIV-1 p24 Antigen, once a test kit was licensed. In 1996, testing of donor blood for HIV p24 antigen was implemented across the United States.

On August 15, 1997, the FDA licensed a combination human T-lymphotropic virus (HTLV)-1/2 test kit for blood donor testing. This new assay

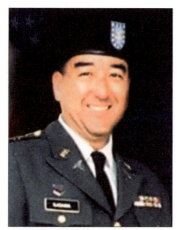

Figure 5-5. Colonel Gary Kagawa. Courtesy of the Army Blood Program Office.

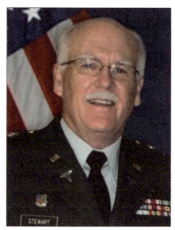

Figure 5-6. Lieutenant Colonel Dennis Stewart. Courtesy of the Army Blood Program Office.

detected antibodies to HTLV-1 and a similar virus, HTLV-2. The following month, on September 16, 1997, the ABPO directed all ABP blood donor centers to begin testing for HTLV-1/2.[26]

The USAREUR blood donor center at Landstuhl, Germany (Figure 5-4), closed its donor testing laboratory and began sending its samples to Ft Hood in March 1999. The primary reasons for this move were increased regulatory requirements, less support from Abbott for testing equipment than in the United States, and staffing concerns. The bulk of the staff for the USAREUR blood donor center came from the 226th Medical Logistics Battalion blood platoon. The soldiers performed very well considering they were constantly pulled between the separate missions of Landstuhl Regional Medical Center and the 226th Medical Logistics Battalion, according to Kathleen Elder's email dated March 2012.

Throughout the late 1990s, the regulatory requirements for blood donor testing began to grow exponentially. The ABP began consolidating testing at four facilities: (1) Ft Knox, (2) Ft Hood, (3) the Armed Services Blood Bank Center, and (4) the Tripler Army Medical Center. Blood donor centers collected donations and sent samples to specified locations to perform testing.

Because the regulatory requirements became so strict for testing facilities, the ABP decided testing would be easier to manage if it were consolidated at a few strategic locations. Therefore, the Camp Memorial Blood Center tested its donor samples and the samples from WRAMC, Dwight D. Eisenhower Army Medical Center, and the Womack Army Medical Center. Ft Hood tested its donor samples as well as those of Brooke Army Medical Center, William Beaumont Army Medical Center, Landstuhl Regional Medical Center, Sigonella, Naples, Rota, Great Lakes, and Camp Lejeune. Tripler Army Medical Center and the Armed Services Blood Bank Center tested only their own samples.

Colonel Richard Brown left the ABPO in the summer of 1997 and became the chief of clinical support services at the Academy of Health Sciences at the AMEDD Center & School. Colonel Gary Kagawa (Figure 5-5) (BBF class of '81–82) replaced Brown, serving until 2000. As the new director, Army Blood Program, Kagawa was instrumental in bringing nucleic acid testing (NAT) to the blood donor testing battery. NAT detects the RNA or DNA of a virus, or other microorganisms, in a sample from an infected person. This test added safety to the blood inventory by significantly shortening, but not eliminating, the window period—the time from when a patient was first infected to when the presence of a virus can be detected. This window period also explains why donor screening questions are still a critical item in blood safety. The new testing methodology could reduce the HIV-1 window period by 6 to 11 days and the HCV window by 59 days.[27] The first NAT for HIV-1 and HCV was not licensed and had to be implemented under an investigational new drug protocol. This marked the first time the ABP blood donor centers had to perform donor testing using an FDA unlicensed test methodology. There was also a debate within the US blood industry on whether single-donor samples or mini-pooled donor samples were the best approach to testing. Those who favored single-donor testing were concerned about diluting the virus titer in a sample below the detectable threshold of the assay when the samples were pooled.

The ABP believed that single-donor testing was the best approach and partnered with Gen-Probe for single-donor testing using its investigational new drug protocol; all samples collected fell under the auspices of BAMC's institutional review board protocol. Because this was an unlicensed test, the protocol required two consent forms: (1) the initial blood donation form and (2) the followup evaluation form. Only donors agreeing to participate in the study by signing the initial blood donation consent form were allowed to donate. Each blood donor center was responsible for encouraging donors to participate in the followup study. On April 17, 2000, ABP Policy Letter 4-17-00[28] provided guidance to ABP donor centers on the implementation of single-donor NAT testing. The Blood Bank Center at Ft Hood, under the direction of Lieutenant Colonel Noel Webster, implemented the test in February 2000. The Ft Hood center was the first blood bank in the United States to perform single-donor NAT testing. The Tripler Army Medical Center and the Camp Memorial Blood Center implemented the test in August 2000. Only three of the four blood donor centers that tested samples established NAT labs. The Armed Services Blood Bank Center at Ft Lewis did not test samples because of space issues.

Lieutenant Colonel Dennis Stewart (Figure 5-6) (BBF class of '89–90) replaced Kagawa as the director of the ABP in 2000. Although serving in this position for a little less than a year, Steward was instrumental in deploying the

Theater-DBSS to the frozen blood depots in Korea—Camp Carroll and Camp Humphreys. These camps were the locations in Korea where frozen blood was kept as part of the healthcare strategy if hostilities on the Korean peninsula began again. Frozen blood would be used until blood donor centers in the continental United States could increase collections and begin shipping fresh liquid blood to Korea, according to Kathleen Elder's email dated January 2012.

INFORMATION MANAGEMENT AND A FORMAL QUALITY ASSURANCE PROGRAM

With the rapid growth of healthcare information systems in the 1990s, the military blood programs continued to pursue efficient ways to electronically capture records and information from the blood donor centers and transfusion services. The Defense Blood Management Information System developed by Colonel Platte and other ASBP leaders in the late 1980s was never fielded to the sites. In 1991, blood bank officers from the three services joined with the Defense Medical Logistics Standard Support office and began development on a new blood program computer system, the Defense Blood Standard System (DBSS). Major Mike Stanton and Lieutenant Colonel Lloyd Lippert (BBF class of '74–75) served as the ABP project managers for this effort. The Camp Memorial Blood Center at Ft Knox served as a beta test site in 1993, and the new system was first deployed to military transfusion services and blood donor centers in 1994. The DBSS was a Class II medical device regulated by the FDA (the Defense Medical Logistics Standard Support office carried the FDA manufacturer's license). However, over the next 14 years, DBSS remained stagnant as a recordkeeping system, unlike commercial blood bank systems that transitioned into decision-making systems. It was not until 2008 that a concerted effort began to replace DBSS with a commercial blood establishment computer system that could easily be updated and changed as industry requirements evolved.

During the same time, efforts were made to obtain FDA approval for automated print-on-demand labels in black and white—not color—as the CFR required. This effort laid the groundwork for the future label printing systems, according to Colonel (Retired) Richard Brown's email dated June 2014.

In 1994, Colonel Brown foresaw the additional regulations that would be required when the FDA's quality assurance guidance became effective, and he wanted to have the program on the most solid footing possible when the new regulations became effective. He knew that a quality assurance position was needed for standardization, consolidation, and consistency within the ABP, and he did not want the program to risk falling under an FDA consent decree. Initially, he intended to use the quality assurance position as a mentoring assignment for younger blood bank officers. Because there were simply not enough blood bank officers to meet all the operational requirements, Colonel Brown had a young clinical laboratory officer, Captain Sheryl Dunn (later, BBF class of '95–96), assume a quality assurance coordinator position in June 1994. However, Colonel Brown soon realized that the position had to be civilianized for the sake of continuity. He created and established a civilian quality assurance manager position to execute and manage regulatory compliance with the FDA guidance. Kathleen Elder (Figure 5-7) became the quality assurance manager for the ABP in September 1995. Colonel Brown and Ms. Elder began holding MEDCOM-wide current good manufacturing practices workshops. They conducted regular facility audits and published reports for senior leadership's awareness so that commanders, who oversaw the donor centers and transfusion services, and their staff could help provide resources or needed corrections.

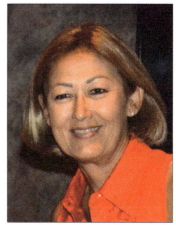

Figure 5-7. Ms. Kathleen "Kathy" Elder. Courtesy of the Army Blood Program Office.

Colonel Brown and Ms. Elder also started to make inroads into standardizing operating procedures. Standardizing procedures and reducing variance were necessary with the emphasis on a "one license, one standard operating procedure" position. The first big effort was standardizing the blood donation record (DD Form 572) and its accompanying standard operating procedure across the Army. Colonel Brown and Ms. Elder worked with the FDA, establishing trust between the FDA and ABP, according to Colonel (Retired) Richard Brown's email dated June 2014.

An August 15, 1996, ABP memorandum directed all ABP facilities to implement the quality assurance program and self-assessment plan.[29] Lieutenant Colonel Dave Miller, chief of blood services at Brooke Army Medical Center, worked with Ms. Elder to develop the template that all ABP facilities used, according to Kathleen Elder's email dated July 2011.

SUMMARY

The decade of the 1990s was very demanding. New testing requirements and an emphasis on a formal quality assurance program drove the ABP to quickly adopt higher standards of safety and quality in the blood supply. ABP leaders, soldiers, and civilian staff were extremely busy, but the outcome was a premier program within the US blood industry.

REFERENCES

1. Allen TB, Berry FC, Polmar, N. *War in the Gulf*. Atlanta, GA: Turner Publishing; 1991.
2. Brinkerhoff, JR, Silva, T, Seitz J. *United States Army Reserve in Operation Desert Storm—Reservists of the Army Medical Department*. Washington, DC: Department of the Army; 1993.
3. Hess JR, Thomas, MJ. Blood use in war and disaster: lessons from the past century. *Transfusion*. 2003;43:1622–1633.
4. US Department of the Army. *Relocation of the Armed Services Blood Bank Center (ASBBC) Fort Ord, CA, to Fort Lewis, WA*. Fort Sam Houston, TX: DA, Health Services Command. Staffing packet, April 23, 1993.
5. Oland DD, Hogan DH Jr. *Department of the Army Historical Summary Fiscal Year 1992*. Center of Military History. Washington, DC: Department of the Army; 2001. http://www.history.army.mil/books/DAHSUM/1992/ch06.htm. Accessed May 17, 2016.
6. US Army Medical Department. Establishment of US Army Medical Command. http://history.amedd.army.mil/orgnztnlhistories/estabmedcmmnd.html. Modified July 9, 2009. Accessed July 21, 2014.
7. 21 CFR, Part 211. *Current Good Manufacturing Practices*. Washington, DC.
8. 21 CFR, Part 600. *Biological Products*. Washington, DC.
9. US Department of Defense. *Medical Readiness Strategic Plan 1995–2001*. http://www.dtic.mil/dtic/tr/fulltext/u2/a402666.pdf. Accessed April 21, 2017.
10. US Department of Defense. *DoD 5136.1-P, Medical Readiness Strategic Plan (MRSP) 1998–2004*. Fort Sam Houston, TX: US Army Medical Department Center and School; 1998. http://www.dtic.mil/dtic/tr/fulltext/u2/a402675.pdf. Accessed June 1, 2016.
11. US Department of Defense. *Joint Tactics, Techniques, and Procedures for Health Service Logistics Support in Joint Operations*. Washington, DC: DoD; 1997. Joint Publication 4-02.1.
12. Simmons JS, Gentzkow CJ. *Laboratory Methods of the United States Army*. Philadelphia, PA: Department of the Army; 1944.
13. Kendrick DB. *Blood Program in World War II*. Washington, DC: Department of the Army; 1964.
14. Gaydos JC, Cowan DN, Polk AJ, et al. Blood typing errors on US Army identification cards and tags. *Mil Med*. 1988;153(12):618–620.
15. Assistant Secretary of Defense (Health Affairs). *Policy for the Use of ID Tags and ID Cards for Emergency Transfusions at the Second Echelon of Medical Care and the Validation of Those Parameters*. Memorandum for the Secretaries of the Military Departments and Chairman of the Joint Chiefs of Staff, March 28, 1995. Policy 95-005.
16. Armed Services Blood Program Office. *ASBPO Blood Coordinating Committee (ABCC) Minutes 11 June 1998* [addendum]. Falls Church, VA: Department of Defense; July 14, 1998.

17. Richter SS. Laboratory assays for diagnosis and management of Hepatitis C virus infection. *J Clin Microbiol.* 2002;40(12):4407.
18. Food and Drug Administration, Center for Biologics Evaluation and Research (CBER). *Guideline for Quality Assurance in Blood Establishments.* Rockville, MD: FDA; July 1995.
19. US Department of the Army. *Blood Bank Quality Improvement Program (QIP).* Fort Sam Houston, TX: US Army Medical Command. Memorandum, September 27, 1994.
20. 21 USC, Section 301. *Federal Food, Drug, and Cosmetic Act.* Washington, DC: 1938.
21. US Department of the Army. *Managing Food and Drug Administration (FDA) Inspections for Army Blood Banks and Donor Center.* Fort Sam Houston, TX: US Army Medical Command. Memorandum, May 1, 1994.
22. Office of The Surgeon General. *Food and Drug Administration (FDA) Revised Recommendations for Prevention of Human Immunodeficiency Virus (HIV) Transmission by Blood and Blood Products.* Falls Church, VA: Department of the Army. Memorandum, August 18, 1992.
23. Office of The Surgeon General. *Revised Recommendations for Testing Whole Blood, Blood Components, Source Plasma and Source Leukocytes for Antibody to Hepatitis C Encoded Antigen (Anti-HCV).* Falls Church, VA: Department of the Army. Memorandum, November 3, 1993.
24. Headquarters, US Army Medical Command. *Policy for Discontinuance of Alanine Aminotransferase (ALT) Testing for Blood Donations.* Fort Sam Houston, TX: Department of the Army. Memorandum, August 9, 1995.
25. Headquarters, US Army Medical Command. *Infectious Disease Testing Blood Donor Deferral Algorithms and Deferral Codes.* Fort Sam Houston, TX: Department of the Army. Memorandum, December 13, 1995.
26. Headquarters, US Army Medical Command. *Food and Drug Administration (FDA) Guidance for Industry, Donor Screening for Antibodies to Human T-Lymphotropic Virus type II (HTLV-II).* Fort Sam Houston, TX: Department of the Army. Memorandum, September 16, 1997.
27. US Food and Drug Administration. Procleix HIV-1/HCV assay. http://www.fda.gov/BiologicsBloodVaccines/BloodBloodProducts/ApprovedProducts/LicensedProductsBLAs/BloodDonorScreening/InfectiousDisease/ucm092022.htm. Updated July 13, 2010. Accessed October 22, 2014.
28. Headquarters, US Army Medical Command. *Implementation of Nucleic Acid Testing (NAT) Single Donor Testing.* Fort Sam Houston, TX: Department of the Army; April 17, 2000. Policy letter 4-17-00.
29. Headquarters, US Army Medical Command. *Implementation of the Army Blood Bank Quality Program and Blood Bank Self-Assessment Plan.* Fort Sam Houston, TX: Department of the Army. Memorandum, August 15, 1996.

DEPARTMENT OF THE ARMY
HEADQUARTERS, UNITED STATES ARMY HEALTH SERVICES COMMAND
Fort Sam Houston, Texas 78234-6000

HSC BLOOD PROGRAM ACTIVITY
IDENTIFICATION NUMBERS

BLOOD PROGRAM MTF	BLOOD BAG UNIT NUMBERS	FDA REG NO.	FDA LIC NO.
1. FT BELVOIR	100-101	1177704	
2. FT BENNING	102-115	1044594	0611-010
3. FT BLISS (WBAMC)	116-135	1677436	0611-004
FT BLISS DONOR CTR		1677433	
4. FT BRAGG	136-148	1044593	0611-018
5. FT CAMPBELL	149-156	1045250	
6. FT CARSON	157-160	1777440	0611-015
7. FT DEVENS	161-166	1270000	
8. FT DIX	167-175	2242649	0611-011
9. FT EUSTIS	176-177	1177705	
10. FT GORDON (DDEAMC)	178-186	1077442	0611-005
11. FT HOOD (TBBC)	187-198	1625834	0611-013
DARNALL TRANS SVC		1629552	
12. FT HUACHUCA	199-200	2077716	
13. FT JACKSON	201-214	1045326	0611-017
14. FT KNOX (CMBC)	215-225	1077435	0611-008
	387-389		
IRELAND TRANS SVC		1046965	
15. FT LEE	226-230	1177703	
16. FT LEWIS (MAMC)	231-240	3077441	0611-007
17. FT MCCLELLAN	241-245	1077014	0611-020
18. FT MEADE	246-247	1177706	

Attachment 5-1.

19. FT ORD (ASBBC) HAYES ACH TRANS SVC	248-255	2977439 TBD **	0611-012
20. FT POLK	256-263	2377702	0611-022
21. FT RILEY	264-267	1978005	0611-016
22. FT RUCKER	268-270	1045324	
23. FT SAM HOUSTON (BAMC)	271-279	1677437	0611-001
24. FT SILL	280-290	1626236	[0611-019]*
25. FT STEWART	291-294	1045325	
26. FT WAINWRIGHT	295-299	3019419	0611-021
27. FT LEONARD WOOD	300-313	1978003	0611-014
28. TRIPLER AMC	314-331	2977443	0611-006
29. FITZSIMONS AMC	364-365 379-381	1777444	0611-003
30. LETTERMAN AMC	366-367	2977434	0611-009
31. WALTER REED AMC	368-369 384-386	1177438	0611-002
32. FT BEN HARRISON	370	1831763	
33. FT IRWIN	371-372	2077796	
34. FT LEAVENWORTH	373	1976039	
35. FT MONMOUTH	374	2242827	
36. REDSTONE ARSENAL	375	1045327	
37. WEST POINT	376	1316137	
38. PANAMA (GORGAS) COCO SOLO	377-378	2677421 2672186	
UNASSGN BLD UNIT ID NO.	390-399		

* FT SILL FDA LIC INACTIVE

** APPLICATION FOR BLOOD ESTABLISHMENT REGISTRATION IN PROGRESS

Attachment 5-1. Continued

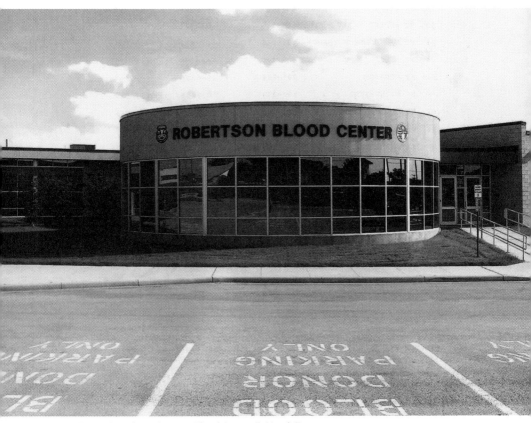
Figure 6-3. The Robertson Blood Center, Ft Hood, Texas.
Courtesy of the Robertson Blood Center.

CHAPTER SIX

Modernizing and Addressing New Challenges: 2000s

In the new century, the Army Blood Program continued to be restructured while the military engaged in conflicts in Afghanistan and Iraq. Restructuring changed how blood was distributed on the battlefield and also brought about the opening of new blood donor centers (BDCs). This decade played a vital role in shaping the Army Blood Program (ABP) and laid the groundwork for the program as it is structured today.

THE NEW CENTURY OF ARMY BLOOD BANKING

From 2001 to 2005, Colonel Gary Norris (Figure 6-1) (US Army Blood Bank Fellowship [BBF] class of '86–87) was next to serve as the director of the ABP. Norris moved the ABP director position back to the Office of The Surgeon General in Falls Church, Virginia; however, the quality assurance manager and look-back coordinator positions remained at Army Medical Command (MEDCOM).

On August 3, 2001, the new BDC at Ft Hood was dedicated in honor of Major Oswald H. Robertson (Figure 6-2). His experimentation with blood preservation during World War I led to his designation as the father of blood banking. Over 21,571 ft^2 in size, the Robertson Blood Center (Figure 6-3) was the most technically advanced donor center in the DoD. The staff collected from the first donors in the new facility in July 2001.[1]

In 2005, Colonel Norris retired and Colonel Stephen Beardsley (Figure 6-4) (BBF class of '90–91) became the next director of the ABP. As the wars in Afghanistan and Iraq continued, concern developed about the number of severely wounded soldiers receiving fresh whole blood (FWB) obtained in emergency collections on the battlefield. The assistant secretary of defense (health affairs) wanted to ensure that these individuals were monitored at specific intervals after

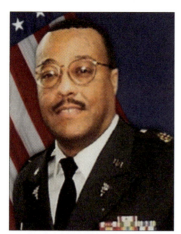

Figure 6-1. Colonel Gary Norris. Courtesy of the Army Blood Program Office.

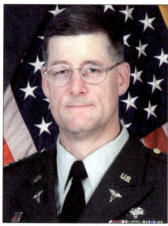

Figure 6-4. Colonel Steve Beardsley. Courtesy of Walter Reed Army Medical Center, Blood Services.

transfusion. In October 2006, a Reserve Component blood bank officer, Lieutenant Colonel Kenneth Davis (Figure 6-5) (later, BBF class of '07–08), was mobilized to augment the Army Blood Program Office. His primary mission was to manage the theater look-back program and follow cases of the patients who had received emergency FWB or plateletpheresis collected in theater. Additionally, Lieutenant Colonel Kenneth Davis assisted Colonel Beardsley in managing the more than 100 reservists supporting the BDCs and distributing the Army quota requirements among the Army BDCs to help eliminate the backlog.

The Ft Benning BDC (Figure 6-6) was established as a result of the relocation of the armor school from Ft Knox to Ft Benning, another training installation. Due to base realignment and closure, the Camp Memorial Blood Center officially closed in October 2007. Lieutenant Colonel Emmett Gourdine served as its last director. However, blood collections continued through 2008 at Ft Knox as a satellite collection facility for the BDC at the Womack Army Medical Center at Ft Bragg. At Ft Benning, a temporary building was constructed in March 2007 to house processing, manufacturing, and distribution sections. One hundred percent of the blood collected at Ft Benning was obtained via mobile blood drives. By February 2008, the Ft Benning BDC had opened its doors as the newest center in the ABP.[2]

With the closure of the Camp Memorial Blood Center, blood donor testing previously performed there was transitioned to Robertson Blood Center at Ft Hood (Figure 6-7). It was also during this time that blood donor testing at the Armed Services Blood Bank Center, Ft Lewis, was discontinued and moved to the Robertson Blood Center, leaving only the Robertson Blood Center and the Tripler Army Medical Center as testing facilities for the ABP.

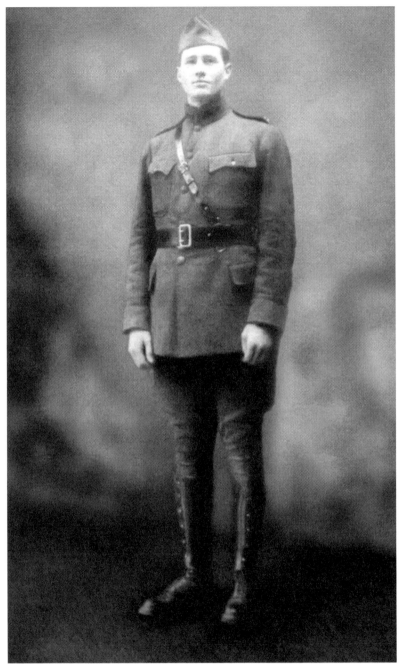

Figure 6-2. Framed photo of Captain Oswald H. Robertson on displayed in the rotunda of the Robertson Blood Center, Ft Hood, Texas. Courtesy of the Robertson Blood Center.

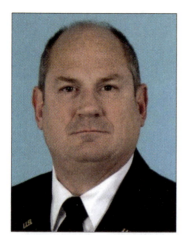

Figure 6-5. Lieutenant Colonel Kenneth Davis, US Army Reserves. In October 2006, Lieutenant Colonel Davis was mobilized to augment the Army Blood Program Office. He quickly proved to be an invaluable asset to the office. Courtesy of Colonel (Ret) Kenneth Davis.

In October 2007, the Armed Services Blood Bank Center–Pacific Northwest moved out of the Madigan Army Medical Center building and into a renovated facility located in the old Madigan hospital, just a few block east of the current medical center.[3] Madigan's commander, Brigadier General Shelia Baxter; outgoing director Lieutenant Colonel Robin Whitacre (BBF class of '98–99); and incoming director Major Angel Colon (BBF class of '01–02) cut the ribbon during the grand opening ceremony (Figure 6-8).

In 2008, after serving as the director of the ABP from 2005 to 2008, Colonel Beardsley returned to Walter Reed Army Medical Center and remained there as its chief of blood services, education program director, and interim laboratory manager until the medical center officially closed on July 27, 2011. At that time, the facility merged with the National Naval Medical Center in Bethesda, Maryland, where it currently exists as the Walter Reed National Military Medical Center. With this merger, the BDC at Walter Reed and the transfusion services at Dewitt Army Community Hospital, Ft Belvoir, Virginia, realigned under the Department of the Navy's Food and Drug Administration (FDA) blood establishment license.

Following in Colonel Beardsley's footsteps was Lieutenant Colonel Mike Lopatka (Figure 6-9) (BBF class of '00–01). Although Lieutenant Colonel Lopatka was assigned as an interim director and his tenure was less than a year long before his retirement, the ABP remained busy. Lieutenant Colonel Lopatka attended many months of meetings and discussions to gain approval for the military blood program to obtain a commercial blood computer system. The Department of Defense awarded a contract to ThunderCat Technology (Reston, VA) to provide an enterprise blood management system across the Military Health System. Mediware Information Systems (Lenexa, KS) developed LifeTrak Donor and HCLL Transfusion software. Both software systems are 510(k) cleared as approved medical devices by the FDA. The contact for LifeTrak was awarded in September 2010 and the contract for HCLL was awarded few months later in March 2011.

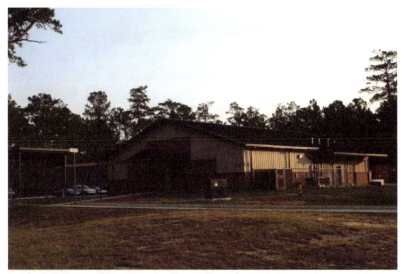

Figure 6-6. The initial blood donor center building on Ft Benning. Courtesy of the Sullivan Memorial Blood Center, Ft Benning, Georgia.

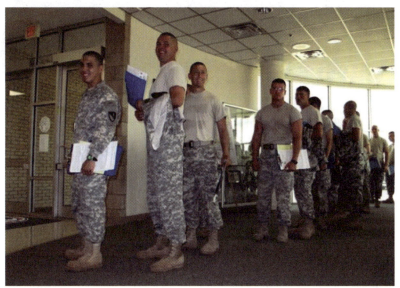

Figure 6-7. Soldiers line up to donate at the Robertson Blood Center. Courtesy of the Robertson Blood Center, Ft Hood, Texas.

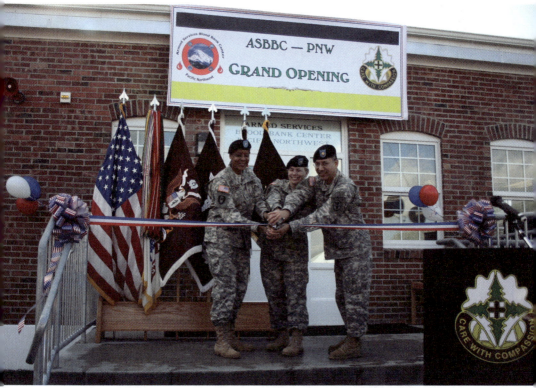

Figure 6-8. The grand opening of the new location for the Armed Services Blood Bank Center–Pacific Northwest (ASBBC–PNW) with Brigadier General Sheila Baxter as presiding officer, along with Lieutenant Colonel Robin Whitacre and Major Angel Colon. This was a renovated area in the old Madigan hospital on Ft Lewis. Courtesy of the Army Blood Program Office.

NEW QUALITY AND PERFORMANCE INITIATIVES

Toward the end of his tenure, Colonel Norris established a metrics program that helped the ABP leadership gauge how well the program and individual facilities performed. ABP Policy Letter 2004-09-02 provided implementation guidance for the program to all ABP BDCs and transfusion services.[4]

As a means to increase quality through eliminating waste and improving processes, Colonel Noel Webster (Figure 6-10) arranged to introduce the ABP and Army Clinical Laboratory Program to the Lean Six Sigma management program in 2003. There were 12 students in the initial Lean Six Sigma class. Colonel Norris selected six blood program officers for the initial training: Lieutenant Colonel Donna Whittaker, Major Robin Whitacre, Major Barbara Bachman (BBF class of '98–99), Captain Jose Quesada (BBF class of '00–01), Major Emmitt Gourdine

(BBF class of '94–95), and Lieutenant Colonel Steve Beardsley. Kathleen Elder also attended the training. When the Department of the Army implemented Lean Six Sigma in 2006, MEDCOM was way ahead of the rest of the Army because of the laboratory program's initiative. MEDCOM won the first-ever Army Lean Six Sigma excellence award for an AR 10-87-level direct-reporting organization. Lieutenant Colonel Whittaker was the first certified master black belt in the MEDCOM and the 12th in the Army. Her first project was reducing the amount of blood that expired on the shelf at Brooke Army Medical Center. Major Bachman finished her requirements to be a certified master black belt in 2015. Major Bachman's first project was to improve the nucleic acid testing turnaround times at the Robertson Blood Center, according to Colonel (Retired) Donna Whittaker's email dated February 2014.

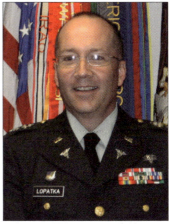

Figure 6-9. Lieutenant Colonel Michael Lopatka. Courtesy of the Armed Services Blood Program Office.

In 1985, the FDA published guidelines that established a standardized labeling system of content and format to reduce errors. The FDA also approved a standardized machine-readable barcoding system, American Blood Commission (ABC) Codabar, a linear barcode symbology developed in 1972 by Pitney Bowes (Stamford, CT), though its use was not a requirement per the 1985 guidance. An April 27, 2005, ABP Policy Letter 2005-04-01 directed all ABP BDCs and transfusion services to migrate to International Society for Blood Transfusion 128 uniform labeling for blood and blood components, replacing American Blood Commission (ABC) Codabar labeling.[5] International Society for Blood Transfusion 128 was a superior bar coding system over Codabar for labeling and identifying blood products. It created a standardized barcoding system which is used in numerous countries around the world. International Society for Blood Transfusion labeling provides a unique identifier for each blood donation allowing

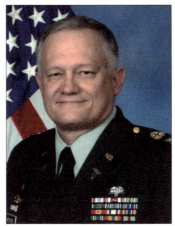

Figure 6-10. Colonel Noel Webster. Courtesy of the Robertson Blood Center, Ft Hood, Texas.

global traceability and trackability. This new system reduced errors and increased patient safety while managing increasingly complex manufacturing requirements. The International Council for Commonality in Blood Banking Automation oversees this universal program through the management of facility assignments, blood product identification, and a global database. Its primary goal has been to implement a standard barcoding system that allows facilities around the world to scan barcodes and determine critical information about blood products. These barcodes would solve long-standing problems such as those encountered by the ABP in Operations Desert Shield and Desert Storm, when military and civilian barcodes did not match.

A major effort by Major Beardsley and Ms. Elder was the continuing standardization of key processes and procedures across all ABP BDCs and transfusion services, to align with Colonel Brown's stance of "one [FDA] license, one standard operating procedure" and improve quality, operational efficiency, and regulatory compliance across the program (Colonel [Ret] R. Brown, email, September 2014). ABP Policy Letter 2006-04-02 standardized the procedure for review and lot release and ensured that the steps involved reviewing documents, labeling products, and releasing these products into inventory were consistent at each facility.[6]

NEW SCREENING, TESTING, AND MANUFACTURING REQUIREMENTS DRIVE ADDITIONAL CHANGES

In January 2000, the ABP notified the FDA that the Korea BDC would no longer collect blood. However, its FDA license was not revoked at the time in case collections came to be needed in the theater. The facility closed because of increased regulatory requirements; unavailability of civilian staff to maintain continuity and competencies; and the uncertainty of whether donors had traveled north of Seoul where *Plasmodium vivax* malaria was endemic, thus disqualifying them from donating blood; according to Kathleen Elder's email dated January 2012.

Another issue impacting the blood industry occurred in March 1996. Ten unusual cases of Creutzfeldt-Jakob disease (CJD) were reported in the United Kingdom. Besides having unusual pathology, all 10 cases involved patients younger than the usual age of onset for CJD. This new condition became known as variant Creutzfeldt-Jakob disease, or vCJD. Scientists believed that vCJD occurred in humans as a result of consuming beef from cows with bovine spongiform encephalopathy (BSE).[7] vCJD results from prions that cause abnormal forms of prion protein, which is most abundant in the brain, leading to brain degeneration. Transmissible spongiform encephalopathy is the name given to a small group of rare diseases, including BSE, which cause neurodegenerative conditions in humans and animals. Other transmissible spongiform encephalopathy examples are chronic wasting disease in deer and elk and scrapies in goats and sheep. The spread of BSE in cattle is believed to have been caused by adding protein supplement from sheep infected with scrapies to the cattle's feed.[8]

In December 1996 the FDA issued a memorandum recommending that blood establishments "quarantine and destroy in-date source plasma, plasma derivatives, and in-date products from donors who were at increased risk for developing CJD or who were subsequently diagnosed with CJD."[9] These donors were also permanently deferred. FDA issued updated guidance to

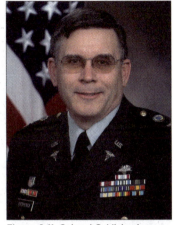

Figure 6-11. Colonel G. Michael Fitzpatrick. Courtesy of the Armed Services Blood Program Office.

the blood industry in November 1999. Recent data showed that the transmission of CJD by blood products was unlikely.[9] However, there were insufficient data to evaluate the risk of transmission of vCJD. Although no documented case of transfusion-associated vCJD existed up to that time, the guidance contained three revised recommendations based on the theoretical risk of transfusion-related transmission[9]:

(1) no longer withdraw plasma derivatives containing plasma from donors with CJD or CJD risk factor;
(2) withdraw all material collected from donors diagnosed with vCJD or suspected vCJD; and
(3) defer donors based on their potential exposure to BSE in the United Kingdom, or injection of insulin made from bovine sources in the United Kingdom.

More than 100 cases of vCJD had been identified by the end of 2001, with the overwhelming majority from the United Kingdom. The number of BSE cases also increased across Europe.

During a meeting in January 2001, the Transmissible Spongiform Encephalopathy Advisory Committee proposed additional deferrals. One sent shockwaves through the military and civilian blood communities: deferring donors who may have been exposed to beef exported from the United Kingdom to military bases in Europe.[10] Colonel G. Michael Fitzpatrick (Figure 6-11), director of the Armed Services Blood Program Office (ASBPO), saw that this deferral would create a potential 25% to 43% loss of military donors, depending on

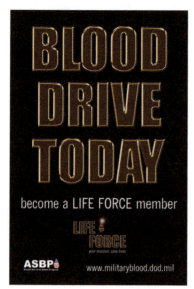

Figure 6-12. Armed Services Blood Program donor recruitment poster using the "Life Force" theme. Courtesy of the Armed Services Blood Program Office.

location and population. He brought this to the attention of Jarrett Clinton, MD, acting assistant secretary of defense (health affairs), and in March 2001, Dr. Clinton asked the ASBPO to develop a plan to manage the forthcoming donor deferral to maintain collections and meet the current requirements. Also in this task was the requirement to develop a long-term strategic plan to meet requirements in an efficient, cost-effective, and regulatory-compliant manner. The strategic plan had to be supported with a business case analysis, plan of action, milestones, and a timeline. Colonel Fitzpatrick directed that a panel convene in April with representation from the three service blood programs. Major Donna Whittaker and Major Ken Pell (BBF class of '93–94) represented the ABP.

A subsequent panel convened just 2 months later, in June, with Lieutenant Colonel Gary Norris and Kathleen Elder representing the Army, and made both short- and long-term recommendations. Short-term recommendations included the following: (a) implement vCJD deferrals concurrently with the civilian sector, (b) develop a media campaign to inform populations at risk, (c) make up the estimated 25% deferral by obtaining donor recruitment and phlebotomy resources (Figures 6-12 to 6-16), and (d) establish an intratheater blood inventory management and distribution system. Long-term recommendations included the following:

- review BDC locations to focus on new recruits and beneficiaries not stationed in Europe,
- optimize current BDC operations (eg, the development of the web-based operational data reporting system released in 2005 replaced the long-used manual DD Form 2555, Blood Bank Operational Report),[10]
- develop dedicated staffing and funding,
- develop a centralized continental US blood management and distribution system (note: this development led to the initiation of a small business innovation research project to provide enhancements to the joint medical asset repository through data analysis and global positioning system inventory display),

- standardize standard operating procedures across the services to reduce redundancy and eliminate duplication,
- pursue 100% leukoreduction through filtration (prions are associated with leukocytes, so this will reduce prions and the risk of transfusion transmission), and
- hire a contractor to conduct the business case analysis to validate the panel's findings.

On June 28, 2001, the Transmissible Spongiform Encephalopathy Advisory Committee met again to consider increased donor deferrals for vCJD risk and weigh the impact of blood shortages. The FDA released draft guidance for deferring individuals who may have been exposed to the agent for vCJD as follows[11]:

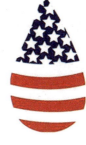

Figure 6-13. This icon was developed as part of the ASPB's marketing efforts to help recruit new donors. Donations had declined due to the loss of many long-time donors when new screening criteria related to vCJD were implemented. One of the first marketing objectives was to establish a "brand" for the enterprise which would be recognized across all three military services. Courtesy of the Armed Services Blood Program Office.

- cumulative travel to or residency in the United Kingdom from 1980 to 1996 for greater than or equal to 3 months,
- DoD personnel stationed in Europe from 1980 to 1990 north of the Alps for a cumulative period greater than or equal to 6 months,
- DoD personnel stationed in Europe from 1980 to 1996 south of the Alps for a cumulative period greater than or equal to 6 months,
- any traveler to or resident of Europe from 1980 to present for a cumulative period of 5 years (applies to DoD personnel after January 1, 1997),
- anyone having received a transfusion of blood or blood products in the United Kingdom since 1980, and
- anyone having taken bovine insulin produced in the United Kingdom since 1980.

Because of the highly mobile nature of the military, especially with the ongoing military operations in the Balkans, trying to determine how long someone was north of the Alps or south of the Alps was going to present a huge quality assurance challenge. For simplicity, these two criteria were combined and grouped into a category that included Europe outside of the United Kingdom.[12] ABP Policy Letter 2001-05 directed donor centers to implement the revised vCJD donor deferral criteria.[13] These new screening requirements deferred many donors because of their military assignments in Europe from 1980 to 1996.

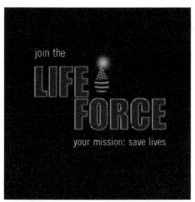

Figure 6-14. The first enterprise-wide donor recruitment marketing campaign was the "Life Force." In May 2006, the Armed Services Blood Program marketing support team won first place (Best Overall Brochure) with the Life Force theme in the Tools of the Trade Awards at the Association of Donor Recruitment Professionals conference. Courtesy of the Armed Services Blood Program Office.

Despite the loss of donors from the donor base, which included many loyal military retirees, the addition of a donor recruiter and additional phlebotomy and technical staff at each BDC, and strategic relocation of BDCs to new installations, monthly blood collections remained higher than pre-2001 collections for years to come.

The potential threat to the blood supply also placed the ASBPO in the position of negotiating a common deferral criterion among the American Red Cross (ARC), members of ABC, AABB, and the FDA. Once the Transmissible Spongiform Encephalopathy Advisory Committee recommendations were made and FDA draft guidance developed, the ARC published draft travel restriction guidelines that would have deferred nearly 75% of the active duty military population and their dependents if they had accompanied the active duty member overseas. The AABB and ABC members endorsed adoption of the less restrictive FDA recommendations. If the ARC had enacted its own more restrictive deferral criteria, the national blood supply—for the first time in history—could have been perceived as safer or less safe depending on its source. Dr. Clinton supported the ASBPO position that this would be an untenable situation if DoD needed to contract blood support from civilian sources. Blood procured for distribution to deployed support facilities must be collected using the same criteria to ensure that all service members receive the same quality of blood.

The FDA and ASBPO were successful in making the case to AABB, ARC, and ABC members that agreement on a national policy that would protect the blood supply from the potential of vCJD transmission and be universally adopted by all blood collection facilities was in the national interest, according to Colonel (Retired) G. Michael Fitzpatrick's email dated July 2014. As had long been a concern, the first case of transfusion-associated vCJD occurred in the United Kingdom in December 2003. The patient developed the disease 6.5 years after receiving red blood cells from a donor who subsequently developed vCJD 3.5 years after donation. Two additional cases in the United Kingdom were identified over the next 2 years. All three cases received non-leukoreduced red blood cells.[14]

Blood screening requirements continued to play an important role in driving technical advances and ABP implementation. From Kagawa's work in the late 1990s on the investigational new drug protocol (IND), the FDA approved nucleic acid testing to screen whole blood donors for HIV and HCV in 2002. ABP Policy Letter 2002-05-02 provided guidance to ABP BDCs on the transition from the IND protocol to the FDA licensed assay.[15] With the implementation of the FDA-licensed nucleic test for HIV-1 and HCV, all blood and blood components collected by ABP donor centers were no longer tested for the HIV-1 p24 antigen. On June 3, 2002, Army blood donor testing facilities transitioned from the nucleic acid test performed under the IND protocol to FDA-licensed Procleix HIV-1/HCV assay for the detection of HIV-1 or HCV, developed by Chiron Corporation (Emeryville, CA).

In the late 1990s and early 2000s, a virus not previously known to exist in the United States emerged as a new concern. Cases of individuals infected with West Nile virus began increasing, and the blood industry quickly became concerned about the possibility of transmission of the virus by transfusion. In 2002, Pealer et al concluded that the virus could be transmitted via blood products and recommended that donors be tested for the virus using nucleic acid amplification.[16] ABP Policy Letter 2003-07-01 provided implementation guidance to all ABP BDCs for single-donor West Nile virus nucleic acid amplification testing under an IND protocol.[17] The Army operated under a Gen-Probe Incorporated (San Diego, CA) IND protocol and all samples collected fell under the auspices of the DoD human subjects institutional review board

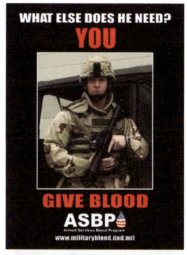

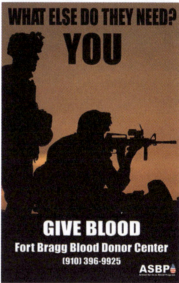

Figures 6-15 and 6-16. "What Else Do They Need — You" recruiting posters. Courtesy of the Armed Services Blood Program Office.

protocol. Lieutenant Colonel Elaine Perry, the director of the Robertson Blood Center, served as the principal investigator for the protocol. Each donor center supported by testing at the Robertson Blood Center was on the protocol as a subprincipal investigator and the protocol was "shared" with the local institutional review boards; it did not require approval, according to Colonel (Retired) Donna Whittaker's email dated June 2014. Like the previous HIV/HCV nucleic acid testing protocol, only donors who signed the initial blood donor consent form could donate, and donor centers were to encourage donors to participate in the followup study. On March 2, 2007, the FDA approved the license supplement for the first fully automated West Nile virus nucleic acid testing for donor screening.

In 2009, after joint decisions by the three deputy surgeons general, the ABP was directed to outsource all blood donor testing. Initially, the deputy surgeons general were looking to get fresher blood to the war zone, but outsourcing quickly turned into a business case analysis. The end result for the ABP was that it was less expensive and more efficient to outsource donor testing. The change was hard to accept because donor testing had been part of the program for so long. However, the benefits of outsourcing became very clear. With the closure of the Tripler donor testing laboratory in October 2010, the ABP was saving more than $4 million annually on testing costs, equipment leases, and maintenance contracts.

In late 2009 and early 2010, the ABP expanded with several other new initiatives such as the incorporation of leukoreduced whole blood collections at Brooke Army Medical Center and the incorporation of plasmapheresis at Eisenhower Army Medical Center, Womack Army Medical Center, Fort Benning, and the Armed Services Blood Bank Center–Pacific Northwest. Tripler served as the pilot site for BloodTrack (Haemonetics; Braintree, MA), a program that provided positive patient identification and improved patient safety.

SEPTEMBER 11, 2001:
THE DAY THAT CHANGED OUR LIVES

On September 11, 2001, the world was shocked when a series of coordinated suicide attacks were launched against the United States. Nineteen al-Qaeda terrorists hijacked four commercial airplanes. American Airlines Flight 11 and United Airlines 175 were flown into the north and south towers of the World Trade Center complex in New York City. American Airlines Flight 77 was flown into the Pentagon (Figure 6-17), and United Airlines Flight 93 crashed into a field in Shanksville, Pennsylvania. Investigators believed that Flight 93 was destined for another target in Washington, DC.[18] Americans were stunned. When the twin towers collapsed, people were in utter disbelief. Not since the Japanese attack on Pearl Harbor had America been attacked on its own soil. Wanting to do something to help victims, citizens by the thousands lined up at neighborhood blood centers

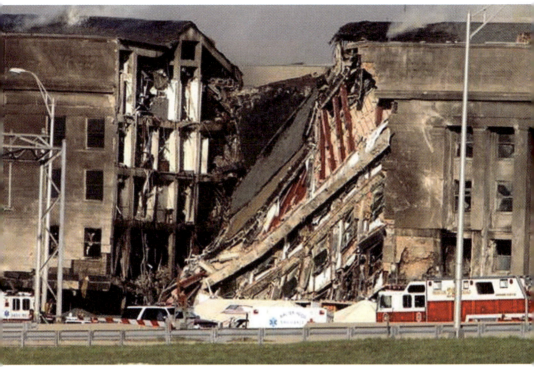

Figure 6-17. Attack on the Pentagon. On September 1, 2001, terrorists flew passenger planes into the World Trade Center and the Pentagon. Another plane destined for a target in Washington, DC, crashed into a field in Pennsylvania. Courtesy of the Army Medical Department Center of History and Heritage.

to donate. However, as the day continued, it sadly became clear there would be few survivors. Yet blood centers continued to take donors, perhaps out of an understanding that Americans needed to feel that they were doing something worthwhile, and perhaps in a sense of duty to country. Thousands of unused units eventually expired on the shelf.

Similar to the civil defense concerns of the 1950s, protection of American citizens from any future military or terrorist attack became an immediate and serious concern. Shortly after the September 11 terrorist attacks, President George W. Bush established the Office of Homeland Security, with former Pennsylvania Governor Tom Ridge in charge, to implement a comprehensive national security strategy to protect the United States. Late the next year the Homeland Security Act of 2002 established the Department of Homeland Security,[19] and Ridge was appointed as its first secretary. During the same time period, the National Defense Authorization Act for Fiscal Year 2003 established the position of assistant secretary defense for homeland defense and America's security affairs.[20] This new directorate became responsible for military activities in support of civil authorities, and security affairs for the Western hemisphere.

The US blood industry was also involved with similar activities. The AABB established the Interorganizational Task Force on Domestic Disasters and Acts of Terrorism in January 2002. ASBPO director Colonel G. Michael Fitzpatrick led the military's part in establishing this group and its initial operating concepts. The AABB coordinated the activities of the task force that included ABC, ARC, Blood Centers of America, and the ASBP. Other governmental agencies represented included the Centers for Disease Control, the FDA, and the Department of Health and Human Services; several healthcare associations and commercial entities also participated. In light of how the blood community handled the events of September 11, the task force's primary goal was to effectively manage the nation's blood supply and ensure accurate and consistent messages to the American public.[21]

Later in 2003, Lieutenant Colonel Ronny Fryar (BBF class of '95–96), ASBPO's deputy director for operations, served as a member on the task force. He was a critical player for the military blood program's developing coordination with Homeland Security and Homeland Defense. As the single military member on the task force, Lieutenant Colonel Fryar served as liaison with the Office of the Command Surgeon, US Northern Command, in developing the blood support plan for Contingency Plan 2002, which guided the US military's support to civil authorities during various crisis scenarios.

Working with Health Affairs, Lieutenant Colonel Fryar reviewed and updated the blood support plan in the National Response Plan, Emergency Support Function 8, Public Health and Medical Services Annex. After participating in the support planning for several national special security events, such as the annual state of the union address, the state funeral for President Ronald Reagan, and the national responses to Hurricane Isabel and Hurricane Katrina, the ASBP's role became clear. The civilian blood centers had, by far, the quantities of blood products available to support these events. In contrast, the ASBP represents only about 1% of the total blood collected in the United States each year. What the military had that the civilian blood groups lacked were tactical vehicles and transportable refrigerators, freezers, and generators; blood support detachments (BSDs) could transport blood to locations where a civilian agency could not. Eventually, the lessons learned from these early support operations played a role in the BSDs being tasked to the CBRNE (chemical, biological, radiological, nuclear, and high-yield explosives) consequence management response force (CCMRF), which later evolved into the defense CBRN response force (DCRF) missions. The DCRF had a smaller structure than the CCMRF and, unlike the CCMRF, had a connection with state authorities.

OPERATIONS ENDURING FREEDOM, IRAQI FREEDOM, AND NEW DAWN

On October 7, 2001, the United States launched Operation Enduring Freedom. Its objectives included the destruction of terrorist training camps and infrastructure within Afghanistan, the capture of al-Qaeda leaders, and the suppression of terrorist activities in Afghanistan. President George W. Bush built an international coalition to join the United States in the fight against terrorism, including the United Kingdom, which participated in an air campaign. The first ground combat action was the battle of Mazar-e Sharif on November 9, 2001.[22]

Blood Requirements for United States Central Command Operations

The ABP was a critical part of the initial medical support to the early combat action in the Middle East. In October 2001, US Central Command (CENTCOM) deployed Lieutenant Colonel Herman Peterson (Figure 6-18) (BBF class of '93–94) to the US Naval Support Activity base in the Kingdom of Bahrain to serve as the joint blood program officer-forward. Lieutenant Colonel Peterson and the blood platoon from the 32nd Medical Logistics Battalion quickly established blood support detachments in Bahrain, Oman, and Djibouti. Lieutenant Mike Bukovitz led the blood supply unit, according to Colonel Richard Gonzales' email dated April 2012.

The first blood supply unit within the Afghanistan operational theater was the 440th BSD (Provisional). Its soldiers came from the blood platoon of the 147th Medical Logistics Battalion at Ft Sam Houston, which was preparing for medical reengineering initiative transformation. Three soldiers (Staff Sergeant Joretha Carodine, Sergeant Richard Krueger, and Sergeant Judy Boutte) deployed to Uzbekistan (Karshi-Khanabad) in February 2002 and joined Major David Reiber (BBF class of '95–96), who deployed directly from Germany in late January 2002. The remaining soldiers joined Lieutenant Colonel Peterson and his unit in Bahrain. During the second rotation of the blood supply unit, Lieutenant Christopher Evans (later, BBF class of '05–06) and soldiers from the recently

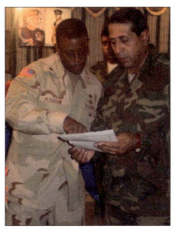

Figure 6-18. Lieutenant Colonel Herman Peterson works with a Jordanian officer during the early part of Operation Enduring Freedom. Courtesy of the Armed Services Blood Program Office.

activated 440th BSD relocated the operation from Karshi-Khanabad to Bagram, Afghanistan. Elements of the 440th also operated small blood supply units in Oman and Djibouti. Between January 2002 and January 2003, the blood supply units distributed more than 5,400 blood products to 20 different United States and coalition medical facilities, according to Lieutenant Colonel (Retired) Dave Reiber's email dated April 2012.

ASBPO significantly increased the services' blood requirement quotas in support of CENTCOM. The total blood requirement quota doubled from 246 units of red blood cells per week to 500 units per week; the Army collected 50% of the total. Although this quota required a significant increase in blood collections, the Army BDCs met the increased requirements by expanding operations without additional personnel, lengthening the workday, and increasing work hours of donor center staff. However, this additional workload, along with maintaining the strict regulatory requirements of the FDA, increased the risk of errors regarding the safety of the blood products at the donor centers; a risk that was deemed acceptable in order to ensure sufficient supplies.

In 2002, the United Nations (UN) Security Council passed Resolution 1441, which called for Iraq to cooperate completely with UN weapon inspectors to verify that it was not in possession of weapons of mass destruction or ballistic missiles.[23] US intelligence agencies claimed that Iraq had attempted to acquire centrifuge tubes for uranium enrichment processes. The UN Monitoring, Verification, and Inspection Commission found no evidence of weapons of mass destruction, but could not verify the accuracy of Iraq's declarations regarding what weapons it possessed. President George W. Bush demanded an end to Iraq's production of weapons of mass destruction and full compliance with the UN Security Council Resolution. President Bush also warned of military actions if the Iraqi government continued to prevent weapons inspections. In the 2003 state of the union address, he said, "…we know that Iraq, in the late 1990s, had several mobile biological weapons labs."[24] On February 5, 2003, Secretary of State Colin Powell appeared before the UN to present American evidence that Iraq was hiding unconventional weapons.[25]

On January 29, 2003, ASBPO tasked the services to again increase their blood requirement quotas, in support of the global war on terrorism. The new quotas, effective on February 3, resulted in a 50% increase in the total service requirements from 500 to 750 units per week of red blood cells, with the Army still providing 50% of the total. Because CENTCOM theater blood requirements had increased beyond the organic expansion capability of Army BDCs, and the requirements appeared to be steadily increasing, the Department of the Army activated and deployed 12 of the 13 reserve component medical support unit (MSU) blood teams to the active duty BDCs to provide personnel augmentation in support of implementing significantly increased blood collections on military

Table 6-1. Reserve Medical Support Units supporting the Army Blood Program in 2003

RC Unit Name	Deployment Site	Number of Personnel
7227 MSU	Ft Leonard Wood, Missouri	22 Assigned 24 Authorized
7233 MSU	Ft Hood, Texas	29 Assigned 44 Authorized
7218 MSU	Ft Knox, Kentucky	24 Assigned 44 Authorized
5501 MSU	Ft Sam Houston, Texas	23 Assigned 24 Authorized
7236 MSU	Ft Bragg, North Carolina	None deployed ISO OIF
7217 MSU	Ft Gordon, Georgia	24 Assigned 24 Authorized
4223 MSU	Ft Bliss, Texas	20 Assigned 24 Authorized
7220 MSU	Oklahoma Blood Institute, Oklahoma	25 Assigned 35 Authorized
7226 MSU	Ft Gordon, Georgia	24 Assigned 24 Authorized
4219 MSU	Ft Bragg, North Carolina and Great Lakes, Illinois	21 Assigned 24 Authorized
6253 MSU	Ft Lewis, Washington–ASBBC-PNW	20 Assigned 44 Authorized
7229 MSU	ASWBPL-West (via Ft Lewis)	17 Assigned 24 Authorized
7223 MSU	ASWBPL-East (via Ft Knox)	17 Assigned 24 Authorized

MSU: Medical Support Unit; ISO: in support of; OIF: Operation Iraqi Freedom; ASBBC-PNW: Armed Services Blood Bank Center–Pacific Northwest; ASWBPL: Armed Services Whole Blood Processing Center

Data source: Army Blood Program Office.

installations (Table 6-1). The one MSU that did not mobilize at the same time as the other units was the 7227th. This unit was aligned to Ft Leonard Wood, which did not have an active BDC at the time.

On February 27, 2003, the ASBPO once again significantly increased the services' blood requirement quotas to meet the increased theater requirements in the CENTCOM area of operations in support of increasing operations in Iraq.

The total service blood requirement quotas increased by approximately 167%, from 750 to 2,000 units of red blood cells per week, with the Army providing 1,000 units per week.

On March 20, 2003, Operation Iraqi Freedom began. General Tommy Franks commanded the US-led coalition. Some 40 other countries participated in the military coalition. Again, the ABP played a critical role in the initial medical support. Captain Robert Gates (later, BBF class of '06–07) led the blood platoon from the 424th Medical Logistics Battalion. Initially, it deployed to Camp Arifjan under Major Robin Whitacre (BBF class of '98–99), the joint blood program officer-forward. Unfortunately, because the 424th was a reserve unit, its equipment was old, did not work, and failed to arrive in theater until late in May, after the 424th blood platoon was at mission completion. The unit linked up with the blood platoon of the 32nd Medical Logistics Battalion. The 32nd's Sergeant First Class Shane Thompson was Captain Gate's noncommissioned officer in charge (NCOIC). The combined units then procured an ISU 96RC (AAR Corporation, Wood Dale, Illinois), an air-transportable, self-contained refrigerated container for storage of temperature-sensitive and perishable items from the 212th Mobile Army Surgical Hospital to conduct forward blood operations under the 30th Medical Brigade. The remainder of the 32nd blood team operated out of Tallil, Iraq. Captain Gates, Sergeant First Class Thompson, and their team followed combat units in the push to Baghdad, traveling with the 591st Medical Logistics Company. Most of the Iraqi military was quickly defeated and Baghdad was occupied on April 9, ending Saddam Hussein's 24-year rule. Captain Gates' blood supply team returned to Kuwait, after turning over forward blood operations to Lieutenant Bautista and the blood platoon of 172nd Medical Logistics Battalion to begin supporting the military occupation period, according to Major (Retired) Robert Gates' email dated May 2012.

CENTCOM blood requirements reached a peak in early April 2003, increasing to 2,200 to 2,225 units of red blood cells per week, with the Army providing approximately 1,100 units per week. By mid-May through June 2003, the total service blood requirement quotas began decreasing to levels of approximately 1,050 to 1,100 units per week, with the Army providing 525 to 550 units per week. The total CENTCOM requirements decreased by approximately 20% of the previous levels, down to 880 units of red blood cells per week, by late August 2003.

On May 1, 2003, while aboard the USS *Abraham Lincoln*, President Bush declared an end of major combat operations and the beginning of the military occupation period. Shortly after the declaration, insurgency attacks began to escalate, carried out by Ba'ath Party loyalists, religious radicals, and Iraqis angered by the occupation.[26] As the number of US casualties and the severity of their injuries increased, the use of emergency FWB collections also increased. FWB has often been used on the battlefield to treat patients with severe hemorrhage or coagulopathy. Because of austere conditions on the battlefield, the long supply lines to support forward deployed medical teams, and the unique storage and shelf life of different blood components, the typical inventory of blood components routinely found in civilian medical centers were not available in deployed military hospitals and forward operating surgical teams.[27] Even though soldiers were routinely screened and immunized for certain diseases such as HIV and hepatitis B, FWB units were not tested for infectious diseases before transfusion, nor did they meet current FDA blood manufacturing requirements. As a result, Health Affairs policy dictated that the products had to be retrospectively tested at an FDA-licensed donor testing laboratory, and recipients of non FDA-compliant blood products had to be notified and followed at 3-, 6-, and 12-month intervals, which quickly created a large workload for the ABP Office. Tracking the recipients once they were evacuated back to the United States and ensuring that they were properly notified and counseled became a huge challenge.

The Reserve Component—A Critical Resource for Blood Program Support

Although combat operations had ceased, it appeared that the operations in Iraq and Afghanistan were turning into long-term engagements. According to Lieutenant Colonel Kenneth Davis in his April 2012 email, Colonel Garry Norris wanted to establish a rotating base of the reserve component MSUs. To do so, four of the 12 deployed units were released from active duty early, during September 2003. Lieutenant Colonel Davis also stated in the same email that because the remaining deployed reserve component MSUs were nearing their demobilization dates in December 2003, 82 volunteers from those units were extended on active duty for an additional year. This strategy both supported current blood requirements and ensured support would be available for extended theater operations if needed. Lieutenant Colonel Davis noted that the current blood requirements still exceeded global war on terrorism blood requirement levels when all 12 reserve components MSUs were initially activated and deployed, but the supporting units were able to meet the mission demands. From late January 2004 through mid-April 2004, the CENTCOM blood requirements increased by 20% to the previous levels of approximately 1,100 total units per week, with the Army BDCs providing 540 units per week.[28]

In the latter part 2004, half of the reservists supporting the ABP were released because of new reductions in quota requirements.[28] At the time, Secretary of Defense Donald Rumsfeld's interpretation of Reserve mobilization authorities impacted MSU blood teams. Secretary Rumsfeld inferred that reservists could only be used for up to 2 years under this call-up and could not be used once the

2-year mark was reached for the remainder of the current mobilization.[29] As a consequence of this interpretation, half the MSU blood teams reached their 2-year mark and were released from active duty in 2005, according to Lieutenant Colonel Kenneth Davis in his email dated April 2012. Lieutenant Colonel Davis also noted in his April 2012 email that to continue support of theater operations, the soldiers released in 2004 were recalled to active duty.

In December 2004, the 7227th MSU blood team from Columbia, Missouri, was activated and deployed to Ft Leonard Wood to establish a new contingency BDC.[30] Ft Leonard Wood was a TRADOC installation whose young training population had little or no reason for deferral and thus was ideal for blood donation.[30] With a staff of just 10 reserve soldiers, Lieutenant Colonel William Walden set up the Ft Leonard Wood Blood Collection Center in Buildings 790 and 791, according to Lieutenant Colonel Kenneth Davis in his email dated April 2012. Because of FDA requirements, the donor center operated as a satellite collection center of Robertson Blood Center, Ft Hood.[30] Administrative control for personnel actions was under the General Leonard Wood Army Community Hospital. After working with the Ft Leonard Wood command teams and post facilities, the 7227th MSU put "needle to arm" in April 2005.[30] Its mission was to collect approximately 100 units per week from four training battalions. The Ft Leonard Wood Blood Collection Center was the only Army BDC whose military staff was 100% percent mobilized Army reservists.[30] Three civilian contractors provided additional support to the center.

Ongoing military operations led to high numbers of emergency FWB transfusion cases by 2006. Approximately 10% of total Americans wounded in action required whole blood transfusions. Trying to ensure proper followup of these cases in accordance with Health Affairs policy (HA Policy 01-020),[31] Colonel Beardsley tasked Lieutenant Colonel Davis to ensure testing interval compliance for non-FDA cases. At the time, the backlog of service members with transfusions who were not notified was determined to be about 450 to 480 personnel. The number of patients transfused with non FDA-compliant products rose to 200 US service members in 2006, then to 209 in 2007, followed by a gradual decline until 2011, when the number rose again and peaked at 278 patients.

In 2006, with all the reserve service members assigned to BDCs having been activated, other areas of concentration and military occupational specialties (71L administration, 42A human resources, 68G patient administration, 68W combat medic, 71B biochemist, 68J medical logistics) were called to fill in the ranks and support the ABP. In 2007, Dr. Robert Gates was appointed as the new secretary of defense, replacing Donald Rumsfeld. According to Lieutenant Colonel Kenneth Davis' email dated April 2012, Dr. Gates reevaluated the interpretation of the regulations pertaining to Presidential Reserve Call-up Authority (10 USC

§ 12304[32]). In Dr. Gates' interpretation, a reservist could be utilized up to 24 consecutive months per mobilization but would be subject to recall.[33] In 2007, the ABP once again brought laboratory technicians back on board from the original 13 reserve MSUs. Using experienced laboratory technicians reduced the training time required to get them into the operational flow. The Army blood program was designated by MEDCOM Mobilization Division as a continuous MEDCOM mission requirement, allowing the program to extend personnel beyond the 1-year period under contingency operations for active duty operational support as volunteers (10 USC § 12301[d][34] orders). This designation enhanced the program's ability to continue performing its mission with minimal reduction in operations resulting from personnel turnover. During 2007, 115 reservists supported the ABP, according to Lieutenant Colonel Kenneth Davis' email dated April 2012.

Changes in duty status for reserve component personnel over the course of the Iraq war made it difficult at times to maintain trained and competent soldiers, a significant risk in a conflict with crucial blood product requirements. When the war in Iraq started, reservists were given temporary-change-of-station orders (per 10 USC § 12301[a][35]) with full per diem and basic allowance for housing based on their home of record. The soldier could ensure his or her family that they would not lose their home, and at the same time, have resources to live off post. In 2008, reserve per diem rates dropped to 55% of the original amount, and eventually were dropped altogether. Soldiers are now extended under a permanent change of station with their housing allowance based on their duty location, or home of record if they resided within 50 miles of their duty location, according to Lieutenant Colonel Kenneth Davis' email dated April 2012.

During 2011 and 2012, reservists ordered to active duty or extended on active duty were involuntarily deactivated and reassigned to the Individual Ready Reserves, interrupting their military schooling as well as complicating their financial and employment arrangements. This reassignment presented challenges in getting volunteer soldiers and officers to extend or begin active duty in support of the ABP.

Improving Hemorrhage Control on the Battlefield

Colonel Norris was faced with another challenge as the war seemed likely to continue. Trauma surgeons at deployed US hospitals requested additional components to treat hemorrhage in patients with massive trauma. Old doctrine was quickly set aside, and the ASBPO and the service blood programs explored new ways to provide better blood support, according to Lieutenant Colonel Kenneth Davis' email dated April 2012.

Lieutenant Maria Johnson and the blood platoon of the 226th Medical Logistics Battalion (Figure 6-19) replaced the 172nd in April 2004. For the first

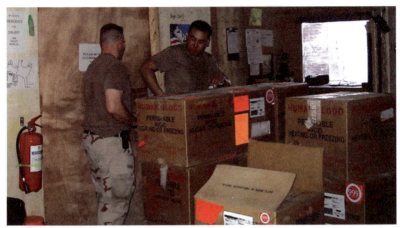

Figure 6-19. Soldiers from the blood platoon, 226th Medical Logistics Battalion, operate the blood support unit in Balad Air Base, Iraq. Courtesy of the Army Blood Program Office.

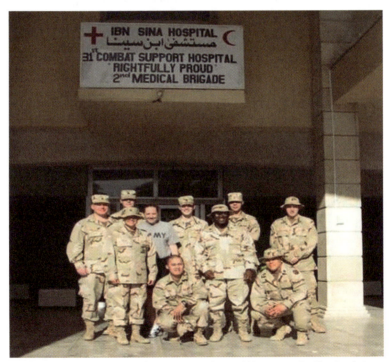

Figure 6-20. Lieutenant Colonel Emmett Gourdine and his team at the 31st Combat Support Hospital during Operation Iraqi Freedom. After their success establishing a plateletpheresis program, this process was used at other units, including those in the Afghanistan Theater. The availability of platelets in theater helped reduce the number of fresh whole blood transfusions and was soon included into the Clinical Practice Guidelines for massive transfusion protocol. Courtesy of the Army Blood Program Office.

time ever, cryoprecipitate was shipped into theater for use at Role 3 medical treatment facilities (Army combat support hospitals and Air Force Expeditionary Medical Support [EMEDS]) in May. The terminology of "Roles of medical care" replaces the previous "Levels of medical care" and integrates with the system most commonly used by our allies. Type AB frozen plasma was pushed forward to Role 2 facilities such as forward surgical teams. Eventually, thawed plasma, maintained for 5 days, was used to minimize the use of crystalloid solutions as a resuscitative fluid.

In late 2004, the Iraq area joint blood program officer, Colonel Webster, briefed the CENTCOM surgeon on the need to have the capability of plateletpheresis in country. He discussed a chapter that he cowrote with Major Charles Bolan, Medical Corps, nearly 9 years earlier,[36] about experiences in Operations Desert Shield and Desert Storm and the need for plateletpheresis. Colonel Webster also used the thesis work of Captain Emmitt Gourdine to prove the need for plateletpheresis in Operation Iraqi Freedom. Interestingly enough, now-Lieutenant Colonel Emmitt Gourdine was serving as the laboratory officer at the field hospital in Baghdad (Figure 6-20) and had been seeking approval for plateletpheresis in country but lacked support. Within 1 week of the brief, the CENTCOM surgeon sent a memo to Colonel Webster stating plateletpheresis was now approved within the Iraq Theater of Operations. Colonel Webster worked closely with Lieutenant Colonel Gourdine to get this process implemented and later assisted Captain Smith, who took his place. Figures 6-21 and 6-22 show the use of the MCS9000 (Haemonetics Manufacturing Inc, Braintree, MA) for platelet collection in theater. This work saved lives and contributed to high casualty survival rates. It is now doctrine and has been added into the tactical and technical procedures for blood detachments. It was used in Afghanistan with great success. With these new initiatives, damage control resuscitation clinical practice guidelines eventually shifted to a 1:1:1 ratio of red cells, frozen plasma, and platelets to treat massively injured soldiers.[37]

Army Blood Program Initiatives

Several additional initiatives affected the Army blood program during Operation Enduring Freedom and Operation Iraqi Freedom. These advances further improved survival rates of wounded military members.

Red Blood Cell Shipping Container

In 2002, Lieutenant Colonel Frank Rentas (BBF class of '91–92), from the Walter Reed Army Institute of Research, led a research team to design a new red blood cell shipping container that would allow four units of red blood cells to be pushed farther onto the battlefield than ever before. They accomplished this by using phase change materials instead of Styrofoam and ice. These are substances

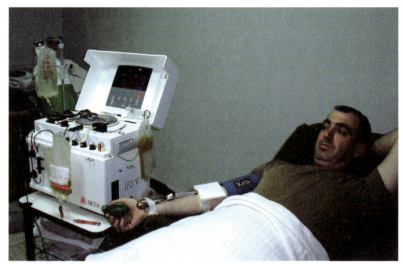

Figure 6-21. Captain Jeff "CajunSuperJeff" Smith donates platelets.

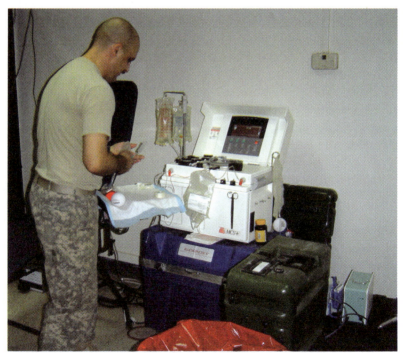

Figure 6-22. A laboratory technician from the 440th Blood Support Detachment in Balad Air Force Base, Iraq, prepares the MCS9000 for a plateletpheresis procedure.
Courtesy of the Army Blood Program Office.

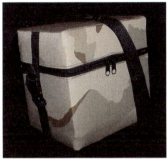

Figure 6-23. [Top] The Golden Hour Container. Courtesy of the Army Blood Program Office.

Figure 6-24. [Middle] A lab tech prepares a unit of red blood cells for shipment in a new Golden Hour Container. Courtesy of the Army Blood Program Office.

Figure 6-25. [Bottom Left] An open Golden Hour Container with red blood cell units packed inside. Courtesy of the Army Blood Program Office.

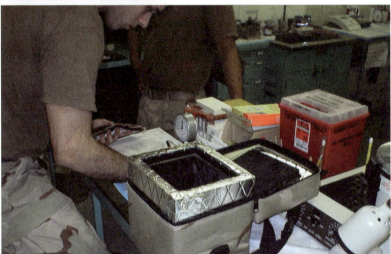

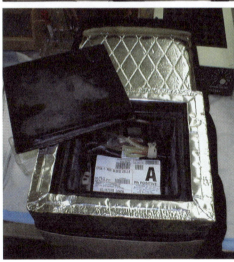

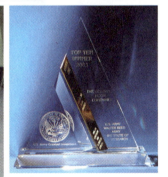

Figure 6-26. [Bottom Right] The Golden Hour Container is a Top Ten Winner for the U.S. Army Greatest Invention Award of 2003. Courtesy of the Army Blood Program Office.

that change phases (solid, liquid, gas) at different temperatures. For the new blood shipping containers, a specific phase change material would be set at a specific temperature before packing the container with blood products. The new "Golden Hour Container," marketed by Minnesota Thermal Science (Baxter, MN), could maintain temperatures for up to 96 hours after being packaged instead of the 48 hours with previous containers (Figures 6-23 to 6-25). This was the first new shipping container placed into use since the development of the Collins box in 1965. In 2003, the "Golden Hour Container" won the Greatest Army Invention Award for that year (Figure 6-26).

Hemostatic Bandages and Improved Tourniquets

In 2002, two new types of hemostatic bandages were developed and put into use. QuikClot, engineered from the mineral zeolite and manufactured by Z-Medica (Wallingford, CT), received approval from the FDA for external use and was fielded by US Special Operations Command and US marines deployed in theater. The HemCon bandage, made of chitosan and manufactured by HemCon Medical Technologies (Portland, OR), was approved by the FDA in 2003 and fielded by the US Army.

From 2003 to 2005, new types of improved tourniquets to control hemorrhaging were developed and deployed to theater. The Combat Application Tourniquet (Composite Resources Inc, Rock Hill, SC) was issued to individual soldiers and the Special Operations Forces—Tactical Tourniquet (Tactical Medical Solutions Inc, Anderson, SC) was recommended as an alternative. Starting April 1, 2005, all new soldiers received training on the new tourniquets.

Type O Frozen Plasma

In February 2005, the ABP BDCs began providing type O frozen plasma to both theaters of operation. Thawed plasma began to be used as a major resuscitative fluid early in 2006.

Hepatitis C Virus Screening

In 2007, as an extension of his blood bank fellowship, Captain Robert Gates researched the different hepatitis C virus (HCV) rapid screening tests to find the best one for use in a deployed setting. Identifying a rapid screening test was important on the battlefield because the seroprevalence of HCV among soldiers was unknown, no vaccine existed, and soldiers were not routinely screened as they were for HIV. An HCV rapid antibody screening test was a risk-mitigating strategy when walking donors were to be used as sources of FWB and plateletpheresis units. The OraQuick HCV rapid test (OraSure Technologies Inc, Bethlehem, PA) was selected for fielding to deployed medical units because of its high sensitivity.[38]

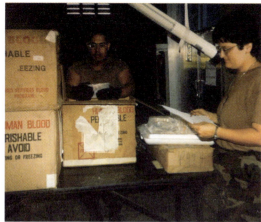

[Top] Operation Uphold Democracy (Haiti) – Major Joanne Daugirda. Courtesy of Major (Ret) Joanne Daugirda.

[Middle] The blood support unit warehouse during Operation Uphold Democracy (Haiti). Courtesy of Major (Ret) Joanne Daugirda.

[Bottom] Blood distribution in the Balkans. Courtesy of the Armed Services Blood Program Office.

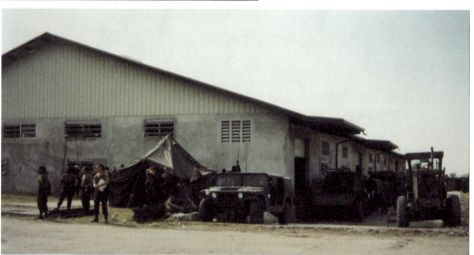

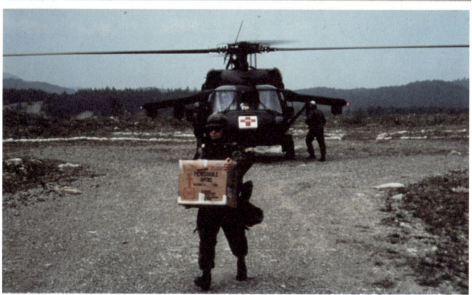

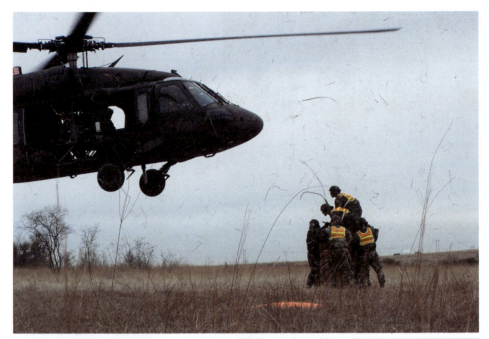

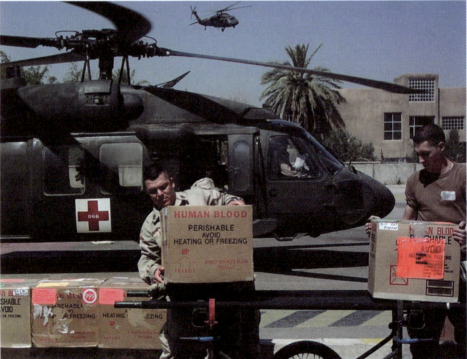

[Top] The 932nd Blood Support Detachment exercise a sling-load by a Blackhawk helicopter at Ft Hood. Courtesy of the Army Blood Program Office.

[Bottom] Blood distribution during Operation Iraqi Freedom. Courtesy of the Armed Services Blood Program Office.

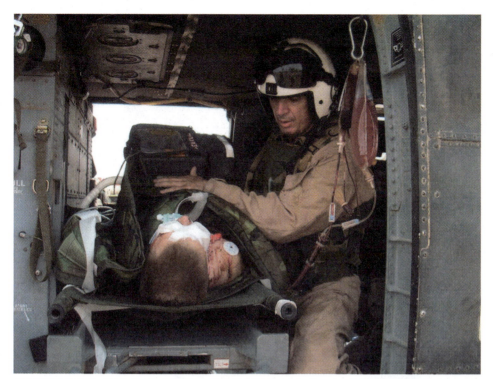

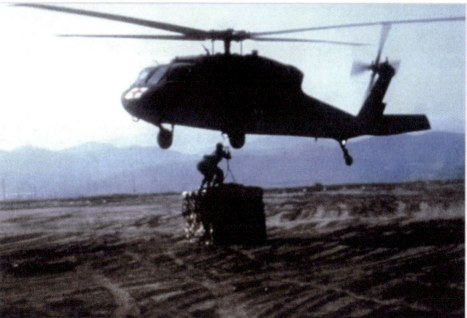

[Top] Blood transfusion during a medical evacuation flight in Operation Iraqi Freedom.
Courtesy of the Armed Services Blood Program Office.

[Bottom] Sling-loading a blood shipment in Afghanistan during Operation Enduring Freedom.
Courtesy of the Army Blood Program Office.

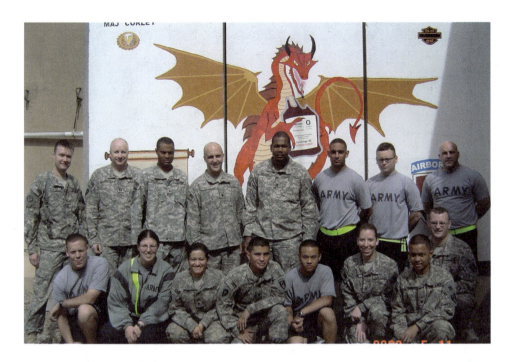

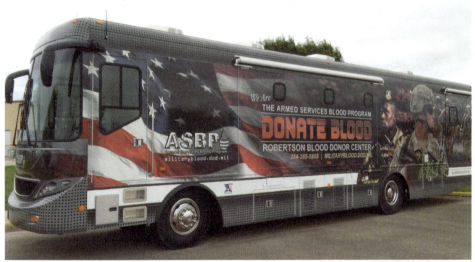

[Top] The 432nd Blood Support Detachment in 2009, commanded by Major Jason Corley. Courtesy of the Army Blood Program Office.

[Bottom] The Ft Hood bloodmobile. Courtesy of the Army Blood Program Office.

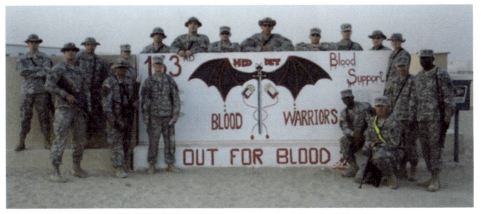

Figure 6-27. The 153rd Blood Support Detachment in Operation Iraqi Freedom—Commander, Major Melanie Sloan. Courtesy of the Army Blood Program Office.

Deglycerolized Red Blood Cells

In August 2008, the 153rd Blood Support Detachment (Figure 6-27) in Balad, Iraq, under the command of Major Melanie Sloan (BBF class of '98–99) and the 440th BSD at Bagram Air Field, Afghanistan, under the command of Major Matt Swingholm (BBF class of '04–05), received training on the ACP215 (Haemonetics Manufacturing Inc, Braintree, MA). The ACP215 is an automated device used to freeze, thaw, and wash red cells (Figure 6-28) and is ideal for helping build strategic blood reserves. They also received training on deglycerolizing frozen red cells (Figure 6-29). These processes were validated later in September. On November 7, 2008, the first deglycerolized unit of red cells frozen using the ACP215 was transfused at the 86th Combat Support Hospital in Baghdad, Iraq. This was the first US transfusion of deglycerolized red blood cells during a hostile conflict since the Vietnam War. As military operations continued in Afghanistan, more and more units of deglycerolized red blood cells were used to treat seriously injured soldiers when blood requirements exceeded the available inventory.

Rapid Blood Typing Kits

As new requirements came out of theater, Colonel Richard Gonzales led the efforts to meet many of them. His work helped identify a rapid test, the ABORhCard, by Micronics, Incorporated (Redmond, WA). The ABORhCard could be used in a deployed setting to quickly determine the blood type of a patient or potential donor, instead of using the patient's identification tags. He also led an effort for a multiplex rapid transfusion transmitted disease diagnostic (RT2D2) product that combined HIV, HBV, and HCV onto a single card for screening all donations collected in theater for emergency FWB or plateletpheresis.

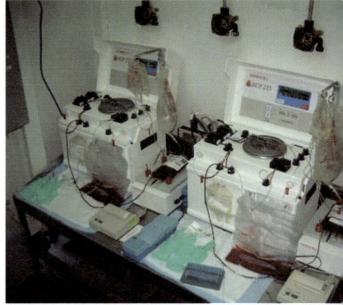

Figure 6-28. The ACP215 is used to deglycerolize frozen red blood cells in a theater of operation. The ACP215 utilizes a "closed system" as opposed to the previous generation technology in the ACP115, which used an "open system." Units deglycerolized on the ACP215 had a shelf life of 14 days. This was a tremendous improvement over the 24-hour shelf life when using the ACP115. Courtesy of the Army Blood Program Office.

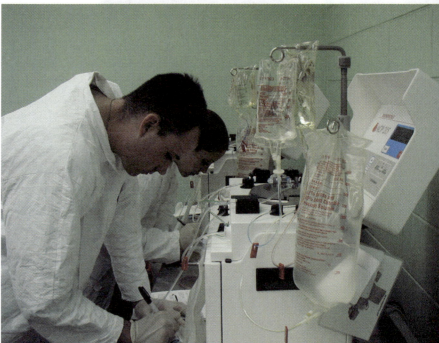

Figure 6-29. Deglycerolizing a frozen red cell unit. Courtesy of the Army Blood Program Office.

Rapid-testing kits became better with time, and two kits are currently approved by the FDA for diagnostic testing. Colonel Gonzales was also involved in the research and development of a freeze-dried plasma product, an extended shelf-life red blood cell storage solution, later marketed as SOLX (Hemerus Medical, LLC, St. Paul, MN), as well as a whole blood pathogen reduction device (WB PRD).

Plateletpheresis in Afghanistan

With the success of the plateletpheresis program in Iraq, the Army sought to establish a program in Afghanistan. In late summer 2006, Lieutenant Ronnie Hill (later, BBF class of 2011–12), commander of the 932nd BSD, ordered three MCS9000 mobile platelet collection systems manufactured by Haemonetics (Braintree, MA), and three platelet incubators. This equipment eventually arrived in theater in January 2007. Lieutenant Hill worked with the logistics staff officer of the 28th Combat Support Hospital to acquire some space within Craig Joint Theater Hospital at Bagram to conduct platelet collections. Major Barbara Bachman (BBF class of 1998–99) and the 932nd BSD (Figures 6-30 and 6-31) collected the first unit of platelets a few months later. Also that same year, military operations in Afghanistan began to change. Major Bachman and her team were tasked to support more customers, especially coalition hospitals. She split her detachment and moved one technician from her team in Bagram to Kandahar.

Expansion of Supported Hospitals in the
US Central Command Area of Interest

The 932nd BSD had already been supporting military hospitals in Herat, Afghanistan, and Salerno, Italy. Soon they supported additional coalition partners in Afghanistan, including the British hospital at Camp Bastion, the Greek hospital outside of Kabul, the Egyptian field hospital in Bagram Air Base (BAF), the Korean hospital in BAF, the German hospital in Mazar-e Sharif, and the Canadian hospital at Kandahar Air Field. The expansion of supported hospitals resulted from increased US presence around these locations and an increase in humanitarian operations. At the time, one reason for supplying coalition hospitals was to have US blood products available for transfusion to US personnel that had been tested for infectious disease according to FDA standards, and to aid in tracking and disposition. Additionally, many coalition hospitals did not have sufficient blood programs and depended on the United States for their blood inventory, according to Captain Ronnie Hill's email dated August 2014. When Major Matt Swingholm and the 440th arrived in theater to replace the 932nd, supply operations continued to grow, adding a Jordanian hospital.

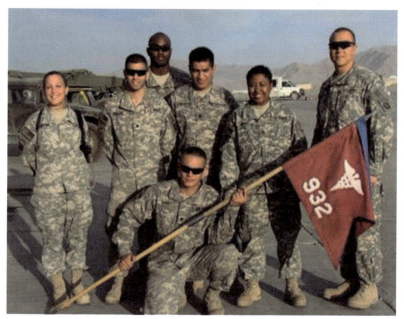

Figure 6-30. Major Barbara Bachman, Commander (far left), and the 932nd Blood Support Detachment. Courtesy of the Army Blood Program Office.

During 2008, the MEDCOM Mobilization Branch published mobilization TDAs (Table of Distribution and Allowances) for the ABP and required the program to start conforming to the TDA. This resulted in releasing soldiers who did not have the required MOS (military occupational specialty) or AOC (area of concentration). One exception was made with an AOC 71B (biochemistry) officer. That same year, the reserves sustained a significant loss of MOS 68K laboratory technicians in troop program units, with numbers falling below 50%. This led the ABP to assess other military occupational specialties to find personnel to fill the ranks. MOS 68W healthcare specialists were incorporated as a suitable replacement for some, but not all, MOS 68K positions. The 68Ws performed donor screening, health assessment, and even phlebotomy procedures, but they were restricted from testing and processing blood products. With the ability of reservists to continue to volunteer and be extended under contingency operations for active duty operational support orders for up to 3 years, the number of involuntarily mobilized reservists was reduced to no more than 12 per year.

The MEDCOM Mobilization Branch decided to designate a derivative unit identification code, DUIC, to designate the unit that would provide replacement reservists to the ABP. Units such as the 7220th, 7218th, 7223rd, 5501st, and the 6252nd were designated each year as the parent unit for new replacements.

Required replacements were reassigned to the designated unit and mobilized to fill specific vacancies. Challenges in managing reserve personnel stemmed from the persistent concept that an MOS 68K laboratory specialists, 71E (clinical laboratory officer), or other military occupational specialty personnel were fully qualified to perform their duties upon arrival to a duty station. As a manufacturer of blood products, the ABP must follow the FDA regulations and the AABB standards. Both require personnel to be trained, assessed for competency, and evaluated periodically to ensure they are capable of performing their job. However, it took time for the newly arriving personnel to be trained on local procedures and for the staff to assess competencies before they could begin to operate in a BDC.

As operations in Afghanistan and Iraq continued, getting fresher blood to theater became a major concern for battlefield surgeons treating severely wounded soldiers. The ABP's new goal was to have blood arrive at the distribution hub located at the Armed Services Whole Blood Processing Laboratory at McGuire AFB 4 days after collection. With process improvements and reduction of redundancies in lot release and labeling procedures, Colonel Ronny Fryar led the Army Blood Program from a low of only 2% of the blood arriving at the Armed Services Whole Blood Processing Laboratory-East on or before day 4 in 2008, to over 99% arriving by then in 2012. This improved process reduced the average age of red cells arriving in theater to between 7 and 8 days, which played a significant role in the treatment of severely injured soldiers.

The End of Combat Operations in Iraq

On August 31, 2010, President Obama declared, "the American combat mission in Iraq has ended. Operation Iraqi Freedom is over, and the Iraqi people now have lead responsibility for the security of their country."[39] The US operation in Iraq changed to Operation New Dawn, in which remaining US troops were designated as advisors in noncombat roles.

As the number of troops in Iraq began to decrease, the last blood unit in Iraq was the 153rd BSD, commanded by Major Evans. In October 2011, the smaller blood distribution mission was given to Captain Paul Randall, lab officer with the 47th Combat Support Hospital. On October 21, 2011, President

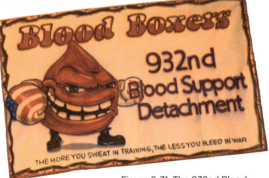

Figure 6-31. The 932nd Blood Support Detachment "Blood Boxers." Courtesy of the Army Blood Program Office.

Obama announced that all US troops would be out of Iraq by the end of the year. On December 15, 2011, Secretary of Defense Leon Panetta officially declared the Iraq war over. The US mission in Iraq would transition once again to a diplomatic mission of the Department of State. ASBPO, under the direction of Colonel Frank Rentas (Figure 6-32), established a memorandum of understanding with the Department of State to provide blood to their diplomatic support hospitals. The amount of blood, however, was very small—approximately 50 to 60 units of red cells per month.

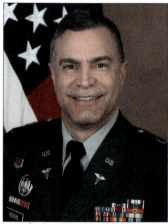

Figure 6-32. Colonel Frank Rentas. Courtesy of the Armed Services Blood Program Office.

Earlier, during an address to the nation on June 22, 2011, President Obama announced his plan to begin withdrawing troops from Afghanistan. Over the next 3 years, American combat forces continued to redeploy; the Afghanistan leadership was to take responsibility for their own security by the end of 2014. However, in April 2012 the Unites States and NATO developed a plan to keep some international forces in theater beyond the end of 2014. Despite this plan, the US-led international security assistance force completed the security transfer to the Afghan National Security Force in June 2013.[40–42]

As 2012 progressed, a new initiative began: transfusing blood under approved theater protocol to critically injured patients on medical evacuation helicopters en route to the next level of medical care. Replacing blood lost through wounds caused by improvised explosive devices or gunshots as quickly as possible has proven invaluable in saving many soldiers' lives. Major Javier Trevino and the staff the 432nd Medical Detachment, Blood Support, helped with training and validating the medical flight staff of the 25th Combat Aviation Brigade. These personnel were trained on topics including basic immunohematology, storage requirements, and management of transfusion reactions. This program became known as the "Vampire Program," and its first mission occurred on June 5, 2012, at Forward Operating Base Edinburgh. By the end of 2012, more than 80 patients had received transfusions on these medical evacuation (MEDEVAC) missions.[43] The Medical Detachment, Blood Support, provided packed red blood cells and frozen plasma to forward medical units such as Army forward surgical teams and Navy forward resuscitative surgical systems. MEDEVAC groups did not maintain their own refrigerators for blood storage so those co-located on these forward operating bases drew their packed red blood cells, and sometimes thawed plasma

Table 6-2. Blood products shipped into the Central Command Area of Responsibility from October 2001 through mid-July 2014

Red Blood Cells	Frozen Plasma	Cryoprecipitate	Frozen Red Cells
422,238 units	172,882 units	41,872 units	3,895 units

Data source: Armed Services Blood Program Office.

for upcoming missions from the local medical element supply. Depending on the location, a few of the MEDEVAC groups, such as the ones at Kandahar and Bagram, drew packed red blood cells directly from the Medical Detachment, Blood Support. Golden hour containers, developed in 2002–2003, were used to transport the blood products on the aircraft.

During the 932nd's 2013–2014 deployment, the number of medical facilities the unit sustained with blood products and support decreased from 40 to 30 in just a 9-month period, while the MEDEVAC groups in the Vampire Program increased from 4 to 11, including three CASEVAC (non-medical aircraft) according to Captain Ronnie Hill's email dated August 2014. CASEVAC is an important patient movement option during hostilities. Injured soldiers can be evacuated on any available non-medical vehicle to quickly get them to medical care, especially when there is no time to wait for MEDEVAC. The use of blood products to save lives during CASEVAC highlights the flexibility of military resources and the need for widely distributed and readily available blood products.

As of April 2016, flight medics, registered nurses, physicians, and physician assistants have been trained on the indications of blood transfusions, administration of blood products (which consists of Group O red blood cells and Group A thawed plasma), and recognition of transfusion reactions. Refamiliarization training occurs every three months. All transfusion data, including physician order, is captured in the patient's medical record and in TMDS.[44]

Thousands of blood products were shipped to the Armed Services Whole Blood Processing Laboratory–East in support of CENTCOM requirements from October 2001 through mid-July 2014, with the Army providing 50% of these products (Table 6-2). Through May 2014, more than 333,000 blood products had been transfused in the CENTCOM area of responsibility (Tables 6-3 to 6-6). There were many officers and noncommissioned officers who led the ABP efforts from within the Iraqi and Afghanistan theaters, and Tables 6-7 to 6-10 list many of these key individuals.

Table 6-3. Units of blood transfused, by product and type, through May 2014 in support of Operation Enduring Freedom (excluding USNS *Comfort* data)

Product Type	A Neg	A Pos	B Neg	B Pos	O Neg	O Pos	AB Neg	AB Pos	Unknown	Grand Total
red blood cells	1,728	13,759	720	7,973	9,599	47,077	2	2	4	80,864
fresh frozen plasma	2,800	13,159	1,076	6,651	1,427	7,077	3,049	16,823	4	52,066
cryoprecipitate	1,097	6,075	198	1,186	1,255	6,372	9	32	0	16,224
plateletpheresis*	351	1,998	84	508	370	1,894	33	225	5	5,468
fresh whole blood†	141	1,237	85	501	187	1,670	24	264	29	4,138
deglycerolized red blood cells‡	11	59	0	1	72	765	0	0	0	908
unknown§	0	1	0	0	0	5	0	3	0	9
GRAND TOTAL	6,128	36,288	2,163	16,820	12,910	64,860	3,117	17,349	42	159,677

* collected in theater using MCS9000
† collected in theater under emergency conditions
‡ frozen red blood cells thawed and deglycerolized in theater using the ACP215
§ unable to determine from early disposition records

Data source: Armed Services Blood Program Office.

Table 6-4. Units of blood transfused, by product and type, during Operation Iraqi Freedom from March 2003 through August 2010

Product Type	A Neg	A Pos	B Neg	B Pos	O Neg	O Pos	AB Neg	AB Pos	Unknown	Grand Total
red blood cells	2,210	20,827	0	4	667	11,854	9,577	47,764	1	92,904
fresh frozen plasma*	2,814	15,143	1,766	10,874	1,566	9,958	2,018	10,071	0	54,210
cryoprecipitate	1,090	6,152	25	81	227	1,338	939	4871	0	14,723
plateletpheresis[†]	367	1,921	17	193	55	510	391	2,262	20	5,736
fresh whole blood[‡]	172	1,614	12	124	99	854	304	2,773	17	5,969
deglycerolized red blood cells[§]	0	0	0	0	0	0	0	13	0	13
unknown[⁂]	0	0	0	0	0	0	0	0	0	0
GRAND TOTAL	6,653	45,657	1,820	11,276	2,614	24,514	13,229	67,754	38	173,555

* includes plasma frozen within 24 hours
[†] collected in theater using MCS9000
[‡] collected in theater under emergency conditions
[§] frozen red blood cells thawed and deglycerolized in theater using the ACP215
[⁂] unable to determine from early disposition records

Data source: Armed Services Blood Program Office.

Table 6-5. Central command total units of blood transfused, by product and type, in support of Operations Enduring Freedom and Iraqi Freedom through May 2014 (excluding USNS *Comfort* data)

Product Type	A Neg	A Pos	B Neg	B Pos	O Neg	O Pos	AB Neg	AB Pos	Unknown	Grand Total
red blood cells	3,936	34,586	1,387	19,827	19,175	94,819	2	6	5	173,743
fresh frozen plasma*	5,614	28,302	2,642	16,609	3,445	17,148	4,815	27,697	4	106,276
cryoprecipitate	2,187	12,227	425	2,524	2,194	11,243	34	113	0	30,947
plateletpheresis†	718	3,919	139	1,018	761	4,156	50	418	25	11,204
fresh whole blood‡	313	2,851	184	1,355	491	4,443	36	388	46	10,107
deglycerolized red blood cells§	13	59	0	1	73	800	0	0	0	946
unknown¥	0	1	0	0	0	5	0	3	0	9
GRAND TOTAL	12,781	81,945	4,777	41,334	26,139	132,614	4,937	28,625	80	333,232

* includes plasma frozen within 24 hours
† collected in theater using MCS9000
‡ collected in theater under emergency conditions
§ frozen red blood cells thawed and deglycerolized in theater using the ACP215
¥ unable to determine from early disposition records

Data source: Armed Services Blood Program Office.

Table 6-6. Central Command total units of blood transfused, by product and type, through December 31, 2016*

Product Type	Total # of Products Transfused	Total # of Patients Receiving this Product Type	Average # of Products per Transfused Patient	Low	Mode	Medium	High
red blood cells	178,343	36,431	4.9	1	2	3	137
fresh frozen plasma[†]	109,306	18,940	5.8	1	2	4	124
cryoprecipitate	31,500	3,253	9.7	1	10	10	120
plateletpheresis[‡]	11,534	5,199	2.2	1	1	2	42
Fresh whole blood[§]	10,308	1,745	5.9	1	2	4	61
deglycerolized red blood cells[¥]	946	456	2.1	1	1	2	16
Total # of Products Transfused to all Patients		Total # of Patients Receiving at Least One Unit of Any Product Type	Average # of Products per Transfused Patient	Low	Mode	Medium	High
341,937		40,173	8.5	1	1	3	401

* data compiled from Operations Enduring Freedom, Freedom's Sentinel, Iraqi Freedom, New Dawn, and Inherent Resolve
† includes plasma frozen within 24 hours
‡ collected in theater using MCS9000
§ collected in theater under emergency conditions
¥ frozen red blood cells thawed and deglycerolized in theater using the ACP215

Data source: Army Blood Program Office.

Table 6-7. Joint Blood Program officers (Bahrain and Al Udeid Air Base, Qatar)

CENTCOM JBPO-Forward* (Bahrain)	Date
LTC Herman Peterson	October 2001–March 2002
LTC Richard Gonzales	April 2002–November 2002
MAJ Robin Whitacre	October 2002–May 2003

CENTCOM JBPO-Forward* (AUAB, Qatar)	Date
LTC Audra Taylor	October 2013–April 2014
LTC Melanie Sloan	September 2014–April 2015
LTC Jason Corley	September 2015–April 2016

CENTCOM: Central Command; JBPO: Joint Blood Program Officer; AUAB: Al Udeid Air Base; LTC: Lieutenant Colonel; MAJ: Major

*As Operation Iraqi Freedom began, the Army had two blood support units deployed routinely—one for each theater (Iraq and Afghanistan). The Air Force and Navy filled the CENTCOM JBPO-Forward position. The Army picked up the rotation in late 2013.

Data source: Army Blood Program Office.

Table 6-8. Multinational Force–Iraq and Multinational Corps–Iraq laboratory and blood officers

Multinational Force-Iraq Lab/Blood Officer	Date
COL Noel Webster	August 2004–February 2005
LTC Danny Deuter	February 2005–January 2006
LTC Mike Buckellew	January 2006–July 2006

Multinational Corps-Iraq Lab/Blood Officer	Date
MAJ Paul Mann	March 2008–October 2008

COL: Colonel; LTC: Lieutenant Colonel; MAJ: Major

Data source: Army Blood Program Office.

Table 6-9. Operation Enduring Freedom blood supply units and platoon leaders

OEF Blood Supply Unit (Bahrain)	Unit	Date
LT Mike Bukovitz	Blood Platoon, 32nd Medical Logistics Battalion, Bahrain	November 2001
OEF Blood Supply Units (Afghanistan AO)	**Unit**	**Date**
MAJ David Reiber	440th Blood Support Detachment (Provisional), Uzbekistan	January 2002
LT Chris Evans	440th Blood Support Detachment (Bagram)	August 2002
SSG Gwendolyn McFadden	Blood Platoon 32nd MED LOG BN	February 2003
LT Sam Ismail	Blood Platoon 312th MED LOG BN	May 2004
LT Lionel Lowery	440th Blood Support Detachment	April 2005
LT Ronnie Hill	932nd Blood Support Detachment	April 2006
MAJ Barbara Bachman	932nd Blood Support Detachment	March 2007
MAJ Matthew Swingholm	440th Blood Support Detachment	May 2008
CPT Craig Mester	440th Blood Support Detachment	July 2009
CPT Maria Espiritu	7220th Blood Support Detachment (Reserve unit)	June 2010
CPT Roderick Clayton	4224th Blood Supply Detachment (Reserve unit)	April 2011
MAJ Jose Quesada	440th Medical Detachment, Blood Support	December 2011
MAJ Javier Trevino	432nd Medical Detachment, Blood Support	October 2012
CPT Ronnie Hill	932nd Medical Detachment, Blood Support	July 2013
CPT Peter Martin	379th Blood Support Detachment (Reserve unit)	March 2014
CPT Steven McDaniel	440th Medical Detachment, Blood Support	November 2014

OEF: Operation Enduring Freedom; OFS: Operation Freedom's Sentinel;
AO: area of operations; LT: Lieutenant; MAJ: Major; SSG: Staff Sergeant; CPT: Captain; LTC: Lieutenant Colonel

Data source: Army Blood Program Office.

Table 6-9. Operation Enduring Freedom blood supply units and platoon leaders (continued)

OFS Blood Supply Units (Afghanistan AO)	Unit	Date
CPT Jacquelyn Messenger	153rd Medical Detachment, Blood Support	July 2015
CPT Joseph Cheser III	932nd Medical Detachment, Blood Support	March 2016
LTC Aaron Mascarinas	987th Medical Detachment, Blood Support (National Guard)	November 2016
CPT William Ceballos	432nd Medical Detachment, Blood Support	July 2017

Table 6-10. Operation Iraqi Freedom blood supply units and platoon leaders*

OIF Blood Supply Units (Iraq/Kuwait AO)	Unit	Date
SFC Shane Thompson	Blood Platoon	July 2015
CPT Robert Gates	Blood Platoon, 424th Medical Logistics Battalion–Iraq/Kuwait (Reserve unit)	March 2003
LT Bautista	Blood Platoon, 172nd Medical Logistics Battalion–Iraq	April 2003
LT Maria Johnson	Blood Platoon, 226th Medical Logistics Battalion	April 2004
LT Crista Campos	Blood Platoon 32nd Medical Logistics Battalion	July 2005
LT Maria Farah	Blood Platoon 226th Medical Logistics Battalion	November 2005
CPT Elaine Morrison	Blood Platoon 32nd Medical Logistics Battalion	September 2006
MAJ Melanie Sloan	153rd Blood Support Detachment	November 2007
MAJ Jason Corley	432nd Blood Support Detachment	January 2009
MAJ Teresa Terry	932nd Blood Support Detachment	November 2009
MAJ Chris Evans	153rd Blood Support Detachment	October 2010
CPT Paul Randall	47th Combat Support Hospital	October 2011*

OIF: Operation Iraqi Freedom; AO: area of operations; SFC: Sergeant First Class; CPT: Captain; LT: Lieutenant; MAJ: Major

*As OIF drew down late in 2011, the 47th Combat Support Hospital assumed the role of the blood support unit for the last remaining medical units.

Data source: Army Blood Program Office.

INFORMATION TECHNOLOGY IN THEATER IMPROVES BLOOD MANAGEMENT

Advances in blood management could not have been accomplished as effectively without computerized tracking methods. It was not until the late 1990s that any computer tracking was available. Theater Defense Blood Standard System (Figure 6-33) deployed early in the Bosnian operation, but it proved too difficult to use and staff quickly quit trying. Also, deployed medical treatment facilities had little to no access to standard military messaging programs, such as the global command and control system or the automated message handling system that would have allowed them to transmit traditional ASBP blood reports and blood shipment reports. However, access to the internet and basic email was common and easily accessible by most deployed service members. By the time the Kosovo operation began, electronic spreadsheets were used for inventory management and blood product disposition. These reports were emailed to the Joint Blood Program Office at the US European Command Surgeon's Office on an established schedule.[45]

Early in Operation Iraqi Freedom, Colonel G. Michael Fitzpatrick, director of ASBPO, worked with CENTCOM blood bank officers and other staff to improve the basic tracking and disposition spreadsheet. Individual medical treatment facilities, blood detachments, and the Air Force Blood Transshipment Center emailed their spreadsheets each day to the CENTCOM Joint Blood Program Office. They were then compiled into a single file that was sent to ASBPO. Over time, this spreadsheet grew into a huge file. Staff soon dubbed it the "MOAS" (mother of all spreadsheets).

In 2004, Major Kevin Belanger (BBF class of '96–97) conceptualized a handheld scanner, much like those used by large retailers, to improve blood inventory management. The Telemedicine and Advanced Technology Research Center at Fort Detrick, Maryland, used Major Belanger's concept to develop the blood information program handheld device, which became part of the battlefield medical information system telemedicine device. Major Belanger completed field testing the blood information program with the 440th BSD during 2005–2006 (Figure 6-34). The device, which fits easily into a soldier's pocket, was first deployed into theater with Major Bachman and the 932nd BSD in March 2007. The blood information program handheld device was recognized as one of the Army's greatest inventions in 2004, according to Lieutenant Colonel (Retired) Kevin Belanger's email dated May 2012.

As the complex blood tracking and disposition report continued to grow, so did the frustrations of its users. Not only was its data cumbersome to consolidate and manipulate, but it was also of limited use in analyzing different aspects of the numerous transfusion events. In 2007, ASBPO began working with information

Table 6-11. Proposed new blood product planning factors based upon Operation Enduring Freedom and Operation Iraqi Freedom data through the end of 2009

Blood Product	Current Planning Factor	Planning Factor Based Solely on current WIA*†	Planning Factors Based on current WIA and estimated NBI§¥	Proposed Revised Planning Factor¶
red blood cells	4.0	3.4	2.5	3.0
plateletpheresis	0.04	0.17	0.12	0.15
frozen plasma	0.08	1.86	1.35	1.60
cryoprecipitate	N/A	0.47	0.34	0.40

WIA: wounded in action; NBI: nonbattle injuries

* WIA is 36,462
† planning factor based solely on current WIA (column 3) = number of units transfused per WIA
§ NBI is estimated to be 13,418 (36.8% of the WIA)
¥ planning factor based on current WIA and estimated NBI (column 4) = number of units transfused per WIA and NBI
¶ proposed revised planning factors (column 5) = (column 3 + column 4)/2

Data sources: (1) Table column 2—Armed Services Blood Program. *Joint Blood Program Handbook.* Washington, DC: Departments of the Army, Navy, and Air Force; 1998. Technical Manual 8-227-12/Navy Publication NAVMED P-6530/Air Force Handbook 44-152_IP; (2) Table column 3 and WIA number—Armed Services Blood Program briefing, data current as of December 31, 2009; (3) NBI estimate—Joint Theater Trauma System briefing data for period February 2009 to January 2010; (4) Table column 5—Armed Services Blood Program. *Joint Blood Program Handbook.* Washington, DC: Departments of the Army, Navy, and Air Force; 2011. Technical Manual 8-227-12/Navy Publication NAVMED P-6530/Air Force Handbook 44-152_IP.

technology experts to design an online program that could be used to more easily manage inventories, track dispositions, and send reports. Blood bank officers with recent deployment experience from the different services worked in partnership with engineers and developers to design and test the new program. Eventually, a new blood module with barcode scanning capability was built within a new online program containing medical information from a combat theater, the Theater Medical Data Store. Early in 2011, the Theater Medical Data Store–Blood became operational in theater.

With great successes in treating the wounded and the ability to more effectively analyze transfusion data, ASBPO proposed new blood product planning factors based on transfusion data through December 31, 2009 (Table 6-11). The factors were subsequently approved and published in the *Joint Blood Program Handbook* (TM 8-227-12) on December 1, 2011.[46]

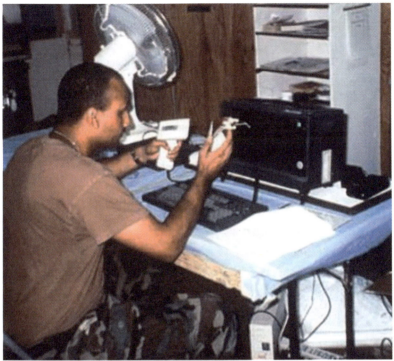

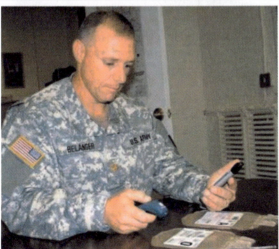

Figure 6-33. [Top] Theater Defense Blood Standard System at the blood support unit in Bosnia. Courtesy of the Army Blood Program Office.

Figure 6-34. [Bottom] Major Kevin Belanger tests the new Blood Information Program (BIP) handheld device. Courtesy of the Army Blood Program Office.

SUMMARY

This decade proved to be as dynamic, if not more so, than the previous. Safety was a continuing focus. "Mad Cow" disease and the impact of prions on the donor population brought new challenges. This added a significant test in meeting blood requirements as the United States entered into new combat operations. And as horrible as war is, new advances in medicine emerged. Survivability on the battlefield greatly improved. But, increased survivability required more blood than in past wars, where many soldiers died before reaching any level of medical care. Finally, advances in information technology have greatly improved healthcare. Systems to collect and study data will ensure that military medicine is even better prepared whenever the next conflict should arise.

REFERENCES

1. History of Robertson Blood Center. US Army Medical Department, Carl R. Darnall Army Medical Center website. https://www.crdamc.amedd.army.mil/robertson-bld-ctr/history.aspx. Updated March 27, 2017. Accessed June 12, 2017.
2. Frigelj M. Ft. Benning, GA blood donor center is open for business! Armed Services Blood Program website. http://www.militaryblood.dod.mil/viewcontent.aspx?con_id_pk=41. Published January 20, 2008. Accessed May 24, 2017.
3. Armed Services Blood Bank Center – Pacific Northwest Official Facebook page. https://www.facebook.com/pg/ASBBCPNW/about/?ref=page_internal. Accessed June 12, 2017.
4. Headquarters, US Army Medical Command. *Implementation of Army Blood Program Metrics*. Fort Sam Houston, TX: Department of the Army; January 10, 2005. Policy letter 2004-09-02.
5. Headquarters, US Army Medical Command. *Implementation of ISBT Code 128 Labeling*. Fort Sam Houston, TX: Department of the Army; April 27, 2005. Policy letter 2005-04-01.
6. Headquarters, US Army Medical Command. *Standardized Army Blood Program Procedure for Review and Lot Release*. Fort Sam Houston, TX: Department of the Army; April 10, 2006. Policy letter 2006-04-02.
7. Will RG, Ironside JW, Zeidler M, et al. A new variant of Creutzfeldt-Jakob disease in the UK. *Lancet*. 1996;347:921–925.
8. Belay ED, Schonberger LB. The public health impact of prion diseases. *Annu Rev Public Health*. 2005;26:191–212.
9. Food and Drug Administration, Center for Biologics Evaluation and Research (CBER). *Guidance for Industry—Revised Preventive Measures to Reduce the Possible Risk of Transmission of Creutzfeldt-Jakob Disease (CJD) and Variant Creutzfeldt-Jakob Disease (vCJD) by Blood and Blood Products*. Rockville, MD: FDA; January 2002.
10. Norris GC. Briefing: ASBP Strategic Planning Information 2001-2005. Army Blood Program Office. May 2005. Located at: Army Blood Program Office share drive.

11. Food and Drug Administration, Center for Biologics Evaluation and Research (CBER). *Draft Guidance for Industry—Revised Preventive Measures to Reduce the Possible Risk of Transmission of Creutzfeldt-Jakob Disease (CJD) and Variant Creutzfeldt-Jakob Disease (vCJD) by Blood and Blood Products.* Rockville, MD: FDA; 2001.
12. Assistant Secretary of Defense (Health Affairs). *DoD Policy on Blood Donor Deferral Criteria for Variant Creutzfeldt-Jakob Disease.* Washington, DC: Department of Defense. Memorandum for the Secretaries of the Military Departments and Chairman of the Joint Chiefs of Staff; August 9, 2001. Policy 01-022.
13. Headquarters, US Army Medical Command. *Revision of Donor Deferral Criteria for variant Creutzfeldt-Jakob Disease (vCJD).* Fort Sam Houston, TX: Department of the Army; August 15, 2001. Policy letter 2001-05.
14. New case of transfusion-associated vCJD in the United Kingdom. *Euro Surveill.* 2006;11:E060209.2.
15. Headquarters, US Army Medical Command. *Implementation of Single Donor Nucleic Acid Test (NAT) Using Chirons' Procleix HIV-1/HCV Assay Licensed by the Food and Drug Administration (FDA).* Fort Sam Houston, TX: Department of the Army; May 29, 2002. Policy letter 2002-05-02.
16. Pealer LN, Marfin AA, Peterson LR, et al. Transmission of West Nile virus through blood transfusion in the United States in 2002. *N Engl J Med.* 2003;349(13):1236–1345.
17. Headquarters, US Army Medical Command. *Implementation of West Nile Virus (WNV) Nucleic Acid Testing (NAT) Single Donor Testing under Investigational New Drug (IND) Protocol.* Fort Sam Houston, TX: Department of the Army; July 28, 2003. Policy letter 2003-07-01.
18. The History Channel website. 9/11 attacks. http://www.history.com/topics/9-11-attacks. Accessed March 7, 2013.
19. Pub L No. 107-296, 116 Stat 2135. Homeland Security Act of 2002. http://www.dhs.gov/homeland-security-act-2002. Updated July 23, 2012. Accessed March 7, 2013.
20. Pub L No. 107-314. National Defense Authorization Act for Fiscal Year 2003. http://www.gpo.gov/fdsys/pkg/PLAW-107publ314/pdf/PLAW-107publ314.pdf. Accessed March 7, 2013.
21. AABB [formerly American Association of Blood Banks] website. AABB Inter-organizational Task Force on Domestic Disasters and Acts of Terrorism. http://www.aabb.org/programs/disasterresponse/Pages/default.aspx#1. Accessed March 7, 2013.
22. Stewart RW. The United States Army in Afghanistan—Operation Enduring Freedom, October 2001–March 2002. CMH pub 70-83-1. http://www.history.army.mil/html/books/070/70-83/cmhPub_70-83.pdf. Published 2004. Accessed May 24, 2017.
23. United Nations Security Council. Resolution 1441 (2002). http://www.un.org/depts/unmovic/documents/1441.pdf. Published November 8, 2002. Accessed March 29, 2013.
24. Washingtonpost.com. Text of President Bush's 2003 State of the Union Address. Published January 28, 2003. Accessed March 29, 2013.

25. ABC News website. Colin Powell on WMD. http://abcnews.go.com/Archives/video/feb-2003-colin-powell-wmd-12802420. Published February 5, 2003. Accessed March 29, 2013.
26. Peace Direct. Iraq: conflict profile. http://www.insightonconflict.org/conflicts/iraq/conflict-profile. Updated March 2014. Accessed October 22, 2014.
27. Kauvar DS, Holcomb JB, Norris GC, et al. Fresh whole blood transfusion: A controversial military practice. *J Trauma.* 2006;61:181–184.
28. Fryar RA. A history of the Army Blood Program: Shaping the way solders received lifesaving blood. United States Military Blood Program Website. http://www.militaryblood.dod.mil/About/army_history.aspx?tb=6. Published 2012. Accessed November 1, 2017.
29. Chapman DP. *Planning for Employment of the Reserve Components: Army Practice, Past and Present.* Arlington, VA: Institute of Land Warfare, Association of the United States Army; 2008: 12–17.
30. Norman C. Army Reserve Soldiers responsible for mission on Fort Leonard Wood. US Military Blood Program website. http://www.militaryblood.dod.mil/viewcontent.aspx?con_id_pk=1700. Published September 26, 2014. Accessed October 4, 2017.
31. US Department of Defense (Health Affairs*). Policy on the Use of Non-US Food and Drug Administration Licensed Blood Products* (01-020). Washington, DC: December 4, 2001.
32. 10 USC, Section 12304. Selected Reserve and certain Individual Ready Reserve members; order to active duty other than during war or national emergency.
33. Davis GP. *A New Operational Reservist for the New Operational Reserve.* Maxwell Air Force Base, AL: Air University, Air Command and Staff College; 2007: 11.
34. 10 USC, Section 12301(d). Reserve components generally.
35. 10 USC, Section 12301(a). Reserve components generally.
36. Bolan CD, Webster NR. Military transfusion practice. In: Zajtchuk R, Grande CM, eds. *Anesthesia and Perioperative Care of the Combat Casualty.* In: Zajtchuk R, Bellamy, RF, eds. *Textbook of Military Medicine.* Washington, DC: Department of the Army, Office of The Surgeon General, Borden Institute; 1995: Chap 15.
37. Rentas F, Lincoln D, Harding A, et al. The Armed Services Blood Program: blood support to combat casualty care 2001 to 2011. *J Trauma Acute Care Surg.* 2102;73:S472–478.
38. O'Connell RJ, Gates RG, Bautista CT, et al. Laboratory evaluation of rapid test kits to detect hepatitis C antibody for use in predonation screening in emergency settings. *Transfusion.* 2013;53:505–517.
39. Lee J. President Obama's address on the end of the combat mission in Iraq. The White House website. http://www.whitehouse.gov/blog/2010/08/31/president-obamas-address-end-combat-mission-iraq. Published August 31, 2010. Accessed August 27, 2014.
40. Remarks by the president on the way forward in Afghanistan. White House website. http://www.whitehouse.gov/the-press-office/2011/06/22/remarks-president-way-forward-afghanistan. Published June 22, 2011. Accessed August 27, 2014.

41. Jaffe G. US says 2014 troop pullout is on track in Afghanistan. *Washington Post* website. http://www.washingtonpost.com/world/national-security/us-allies-and-afghan-government-ready-plan-for-end-of-combat-operations-in-2014/2012/04/18/gIQAX9bZQT_story.html. Published April 18, 2012. Accessed August 27, 2014.
42. North Atlantic Treaty Organization, International Security Assistance Force. Commander ISAF's Afghanistan update, winter 2014. http://www.isaf.nato.int/article/isaf-news/commander-isafs-afghanistan-update-winter-2014.html. Published March 6, 2014. Accessed August 27, 2014.
43. Barker R. Medevac crews in Afghanistan increase en-route care. US Army website. http://www.army.mil/article/93788. Published January 4, 2013. Accessed August 27, 2014.
44. Taylor AL, Corley JB. Theater blood support in the prehospital setting. *US Army Med Dep J*. 2016;April-September:43–47.
45. Fryar RA, Reiber DT. U.S. blood program in Kosovo – The first year. *Society Scope*. Fall 2000;3(2):1.
46. Armed Services Blood Program. *Joint Blood Program Handbook*. Washington, DC: DA; 2011. Technical Manual 8-227-12.

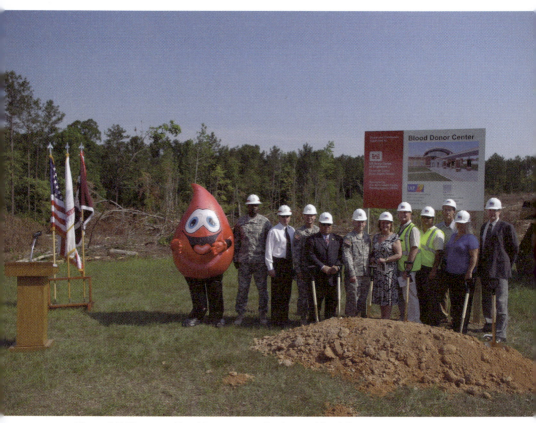

Figure 7-5. The ground breaking ceremony for the new blood donor center building on Ft Benning, Georgia, 23 May, 2011. Colonel Ronny Fryar is joined by installation and Corps of Engineer leaders. Courtesy of the Sullivan Memorial Blood Center, Ft Benning, Georgia.

CHAPTER SEVEN

Today's Army Blood Program

It took decades of work by a large group of influential leaders to shape the Army Blood Program (ABP). From its roots in World War II, through the years of the Vietnam War, the Cold War in the late 1970s and 1980s, and the recent conflicts in the Middle East, the ABP continuously improved the way it collected, stored, shipped, and transfused blood. Today the program continues to mold itself into a leading supplier of blood for service members, retirees, and their families worldwide.

CONTINUED FORWARD MOVEMENT AND STRATEGY ADJUSTMENT

In 2009, the ABP quality assurance program was expanded, and Lieutenant Colonel (Retired) Dave Reiber (Figure 7-1) (US Army Blood Bank Fellowship [BBF] class of '95–96) became the assistant quality assurance manager. Initially, Lieutenant Colonel Reiber assisted Ms. Kathleen Elder in administering the quality assurance program for the ABP, conducting audits and reviewing critical policies and procedures. Lt Colonel Reiber also took the lead on working with the staff at all ABP blood donor centers and transfusion services on standard operating procedures and standardization efforts, including information mapping procedures. He handled many peripheral information technology projects used in the Armed Services Blood Program (ASBP). One of his key projects was the validation of the new International Society for Blood Transfusion labeling software and equipment. He also built and administered the ABP site on Army Knowledge Online, where all of the program's policies and other critical documents and information are maintained. With Lieutenant Colonel Reiber's strong knowledge of computers and information technology systems, he became a leader in the development and deployment of the new commercial blood computer systems that eventually replaced the Defense Blood Standard System.

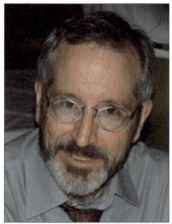

Figure 7-1. Lieutenant Colonel (Ret) David Rieber. Courtesy of the Army Blood Program Office.

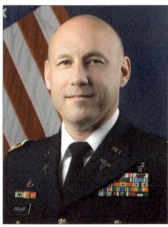

Figure 7-2. Colonel Ronny Fryar. Courtesy of the Army Blood Program Office.

In July 2009, Colonel Ronny Fryar (Figure 7-2) became director of the ABP. Around this time, Brooke Army Medical Center and the Armed Services Blood Bank Center–Europe at Landstuhl, Germany, began sending their blood donor testing to Wilford Hall Medical Center at Lackland Air Force Base, Texas. Other donor centers soon followed, sending their testing to other locations (Table 7-1). Colonel Fryar completed the outsourcing of ABP donor testing. Under his guidance, donor centers established contracts mostly with civilian testing facilities within their regions of operation, in part to help expedite test result turnaround times.

With donor testing outsourced to civilian blood donor testing facilities, Colonel Fryar directed the Robertson Blood Center to take on two new missions: (1) plateletpheresis using the MCS9000 and (2) frozen red blood cell deglycerolization using the ACP215. Both of these pieces of equipment were now standard in field medical equipment sets. Ft Hood began a transformation into a premier predeployment blood program training site, with the Robertson Blood Center as the lead facility. Deploying units and individuals received training on the new plateletpheresis and deglycerolization processes, as well as on other topics such as blood reporting tools, emergency fresh whole blood collection requirements, and rapid screening test for infectious diseases. Units and individuals also coordinated for refresher training on routine transfusion service procedures at the Carl R. Darnall Army Medical Center and blood distribution training from the 932nd Medical Detachment, Blood Support. Eventually, Ft Hood became a one-stop shop for predeployment blood program training.

At the same time, the ASBP Office began looking at the frozen blood program it had restarted in 2005 with the new generation of inventory frozen

Table 7-1. Initial outsourced blood donor testing locations

Blood Donor Center	Testing Location	Testing Began
Brooke Army Medical Center, Texas	Wilford Hall Medical Center, Lackland Air Force Base, Texas	July 2009
Armed Services Blood Bank Center–Europe, Germany		October 2009
Armed Services Blood Bank Center–Pacific Northwest, Washington	Puget Sound Blood Center, Seattle, Washington	October 2009
Tripler Army Medical Center, Hawaii		October 2010
Walter Reed Army Medical Center, Washington, DC.	American Red Cross National Testing Laboratory, Charlotte, North Carolina	November 2009
Dwight D. Eisenhower Army Medical Center, Georgia		January 2010
Womack Army Medical Center, North Carolina		January 2010
Ft Benning Blood Donor Center, Georgia		January 2010
Naval Medical Center Portsmouth, Virginia*		January 2010
Naval Hospital Camp Lejeune, North Carolina*		January 2010
William Beaumont Army Medical Center, Texas	Blood Systems Laboratories, Bedford, Texas (merged with Florida Blood Center to form Creative Testing Solutions [CTS])	November 2009
Robertson Blood Center, Texas		November 2009
Ft Leonard Wood, Missouri		November 2009

* Two Navy blood donor centers joined the contract with the American Red Cross.

Data source: Army Blood Program Office.

with the ACP215. One of the program's key goals was to ensure that inventory did not remain static, failing to keep up with new requirements, as had the previous generation of frozen red cells. The ASBP Office wanted to ensure that new inventory was rotated and used as a supplement to regular red cell inventories at military treatment facilities. The ABP led the way, establishing additional deglycerolization points at the Army Medical Department's remote locations: Landstuhl (Germany), Vicenza (Italy), Tripler (Hawaii), and the Brian Allgood Army Community Hospital/121st Combat Support Hospital in Korea, which represented the largest expansion of the frozen blood program in decades.

From late 2008 and through the next several years, rising healthcare costs, a growing federal deficit, and uncertainty about future budgets impacted many organizations. Colonel Fryar's vision for the ABP was to ensure that the program was business wise, operationally efficient, and always patient focused. To meet these goals, Colonel Fryar and several other senior blood program officers developed and published the *US Army Blood Program—Strategic Plan, 2012–2015*, which contained the following five broad goals[1]:

(1) Foster the development of qualified staff and excellent warfighter medical support.
(2) Improve safety and program efficiencies.
(3) Reduce costs associated with blood collections.
(4) Modernize and standardize the ABP infrastructure.
(5) Communicate with stakeholders to maintain and enhance the reputation of the ABP.

In December 2010, Congress enacted a bill specifying that the policy against homosexuals serving openly in the military would be repealed. The "Don't Ask, Don't Tell" policy remained until President Barack Obama, Secretary of Defense Panetta, and Chairman of the Joint Chiefs of Staff Admiral Mullins certified that its repeal would not harm military readiness. On July 22, 2011, the three presented the certification documents to Congress and set an end date of "Don't Ask, Don't Tell" for September 20, 2011.[2] With the policy officially repealed, the ABP, along with the rest of the ASBP, could now consider retiring the long-standing DD572 (blood donation record) form and implementing the AABB's (formerly the American Association of Blood Banks) Donor History Questionnaire. Previously all high-risk behavior questions were grouped together, based on the deferral period, and donors provided a single "yes" or "no" answer to the entire group. If a donor answered "yes," the donor center staff did not know which specific question it may have been, but the donors were still deferred appropriately. This protected soldiers from career-ending personnel actions during the "Don't Ask, Don't Tell" policy period, but was no longer needed after its repeal. The detailed information provided through use of the AABB Donor History Questionnaire could be used for blood program process improvements and adjustments.

As 2011 ended, the ABP had nine active licensed blood donor centers, one satellite collection facility at Ft Leonard Wood, and 25 registered transfusion services—five that were also part of a hospital blood donor center and therefore registered and licensed (Brooke Army Medical Center, Dwight D. Eisenhower Army Medical Center, Tripler Army Medical Center, William Beaumont Army Medical Center, and Womack Army Medical Center).

During the spring of 2012, the Army surgeon general, Lieutenant General Patricia Horoho, began reorganizing the Office of The Surgeon General and Army Medical Command staff into a general staff system construct. She hired Colonel John Cho to develop the structure. He quickly realized that some critical positions at Medical Command needed to be relocated to the Office of The Surgeon General to improve operational efficiency. At the same time, the Office of The Surgeon General was relocating from the Skyline office complex in Falls Church, Virginia, into the new Defense Health Headquarters in Falls Church. With staff from Health Affairs, Tricare Management Agency, and the three military service surgeon general offices, space was at a premium in the new Defense Health Headquarters facility. As a result, Colonel Cho directed, and the Medical Command chief of staff, Herbert Coley, approved, the relocation of the ABP director and deputy director positions to San Antonio, Texas. After 11 years of the ABP Office being split between San Antonio and the national capitol region, the office was once again consolidated in one location.

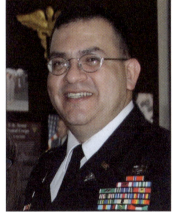

Figure 7-3. Colonel Richard Gonzales. Courtesy of the Army Blood Program Office.

In September 2012 Colonel Richard Gonzales (Figure 7-3) became the next the director of the ABP, as Colonel Fryar moved to Brooke Army Medical Center to serve as the deputy commander for allied health. Colonel Gonzales entered into two major efforts: (1) the ongoing Enterprise Blood Management System acquisition project and (2) the updating of the DD572 donor history questionnaire, incorporating the screening questions of the AABB's questionnaire.

During the latter half of 2012, the ABP, along with the other service blood programs, began to roll out the new full length donor health questionnaire. ABP

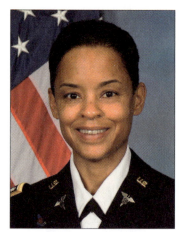

Figure 7-4. Lieutenant Colonel Audra Taylor. Courtesy of Lieutenant Colonel Audra Taylor.

Policy Letter 2012-11-02 set a date of January 1, 2013, for all Army donor centers to implement the new procedure.[3] The policy included several key changes. The time period for variant Creutzfeldt-Jakob disease deferral for Belgium, the Netherlands, and Germany was changed from 1980–1996 to 1980–1990 in accordance with new Food and Drug Administration (FDA) guidance. However, because of the concern about accurate donor information, the Army decided not to implement a reentry protocol for those donors deferred under the previous time period. Another big change was the end of the long-standing practice of directly asking donors questions about high-risk behaviors. Also, staff began to use a much shorter medication deferral list, about one page long, compared to the comprehensive ASBP medication list, which was difficult to keep current. For any medications not on the short list, the donor would be evaluated based on the reason why the medication was prescribed.

In October 2014, Lieutenant Colonel Audra Taylor (Figure 7-4) (BBF class of '03–04) followed the retiring Colonel Gonzales as the next director of the ABP. Lieutenant Colonel Taylor became the first woman to hold this position.

LEVERAGING INFORMATION TECHNOLOGY AND INFORMATION ASSURANCE

US Army Reserve Lieutenant Colonel Ken Davis led the design of a web-based blood management tool in 2010 to facilitate improved communication across all three services, assist in cross-leveling inventories, and reduce blood product expirations. During the first year of the new program, the ASBP saw more than a 14% reduction in purchased blood products and a reduction in red cell expiration of more than 30%. Lieutenant Colonel Reiber leveraged the success of this program and designed a module for the ABP metrics. The new module made it easier for facilities to input their respective site data and allowed management to analyze the data to help shape policy and procedures.

Within the goals of the *US Army Blood Program—Strategic Plan, 2012–2015*, several objectives specified using state-of-the-art information technology.[1] Two blood establishment computer systems by Mediware Information Systems (Lenexa, KS) were acquired to replace the outdated Defense Blood Standard System. These systems were LifeTrak blood donor center software and HCLL transfusion services software. The new software led to a huge project of table and file builds, standard operating procedure development, validation, and training. The ABP worked alongside the ASBPO, the Navy Blood Program, and the Air Force Blood Program in these efforts. The ABP members on the LifeTrak team were Kathy Elder, Dave Reiber, and Todd Cosgrove; Marta Harshbarger and Debbie Van Ronzelen joined Dave Reiber on the HCLL team.

In January 2012, the ABP entered into a lifetime business associate agreement with the AABB to ensure compliance with the Health Insurance Portability and Accountability Act of 1996 and the Health Information Technology for Economic and Clinical Health Act (Title XIII of the American Recovery and Reinvestment Act of 2009) during any audit or accrediting service. The agreement also protected the privacy and security of protected health information.[4]

THE IMPACT OF GLOBAL EMERGING INFECTIOUS DISEASES

Much like the West Nile virus, other diseases have started to cross borders and appear in nonendemic areas because of immigration and increased international travel. Chagas disease, caused by the parasite *Trypanosoma cruzi*, is endemic in Mexico, Central America, and South America. Because Chagas is transmitted by blood, the US blood industry became concerned as cases of the disease appeared in the United States. The FDA recommended that blood donors be tested for *T cruzi* in 1989, but a licensed test was not available until December 2007.[5] In the interim, blood centers identified at-risk donors by using specific questions during the donor interview and health history assessment. The FDA released final guidance on the use of serological tests to reduce the transmission risk of *T cruzi* infection in whole blood and blood components intended for transfusion in December 2010. The document directed implementation of all recommendations within the guidance no later than December 31, 2011.[6] ABP Policy Letter 2011-11-02 directed all Army blood donor centers to implement Chagas testing and to update procedures for donor screening, donor deferral, notification, and look-back processes.[7]

The blood industry continues to monitor many infectious agents that have the potential to affect the safety of the nation's blood supply as some agents emerge in previously nonendemic areas. In 2016, the Zika virus popped onto the US blood industry radar. Early in that year, a child with microcephaly was born from a mother who recently lived in South America. Shortly after that, sexual transmission of the virus became a concern. The blood industry worked fast, initially issuing travel guidelines while a testing assay could be developed. Later in 2016, the blood industry began testing for antibodies to *T cruzi* under the Investigational New Drug program. Looking forward, other infectious agents remain on the radar, including Dengue viruses, *Babesia* species, Chikungunya virus, *Leishmania* species, and *Plasmodium* species.[8]

MODERNIZING FACILITIES

Many new medical treatment facilities and blood centers were programmed in the Army military construction program. New blood donor centers were already under construction or being planned at Ft Benning (Figure 7-5), Ft Bragg, Ft Gordon, Ft Bliss, and Ft Leonard Wood. On September 23, 2010, the Ft Bragg Blood Donor Center moved into its new state-of-the-art facility adjacent to the North Post Exchange and Commissary (Figure 7-6). The Sullivan Blood Center at Ft Benning broke ground on its new facility in March 2011 and opened in July 2012 (Figure 7-7). Under direction of the Health Facility Planning Agency, additional blood center improvements were made. In June 2014, the Kendrick Memorial Blood Center at Ft Gordon moved into a new facility. In April 2015, the blood center at Ft Bliss moved into a newly renovated building. Ft Leonard Wood moved to an improved facility, a renovated dining facility, in 2014.

On July 24, 2012, the new blood donor center at Ft Benning opened and was named after Lieutenant Colonel Eugene R. Sullivan (Figure 7-8). A physician in World War II, Sullivan established a blood collection and distribution system for American forces in the North Africa campaign. The Sullivan Memorial Blood Center has new capabilities compared to the temporary building where it operated since its establishment on Ft Benning in February 2008, including ample room to conduct in-house blood drives and perform apheresis collections.

On June 12, 2014, the staff of the Kendrick Memorial Blood Center moved into a new facility (Figure 7-9). The previous facility, which was more than 20 years old, was an old converted medical clinic whose design was not ideal for collecting blood. The new building allows the staff to conduct more blood drives with significantly fewer challenges than those typically encountered in mobile blood drives in gymnasiums or other buildings on the installation.[9]

On April 23, 2015, William Beaumont Army Medical Center on Ft Bliss, Texas, opened a new facility for their blood donor center. The new facility has more than twice the square footage of the previous facility, and this 7,000 ft^2 building allows a more efficient operations and donor flow.[10]

MAINTAINING AN ACTIVE ROLE IN RESEARCH AND DEVELOPMENT

Colonel Gonzales also ensured that the ABP remained actively involved in research and development efforts for new products and improvements in the safety of the blood supply to support the Army in 2020 and beyond. His efforts

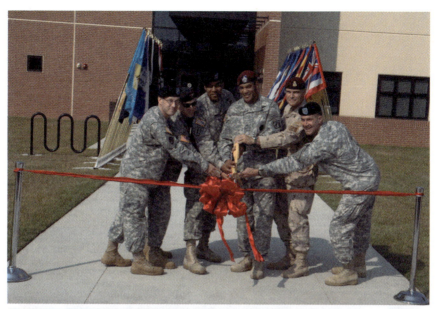

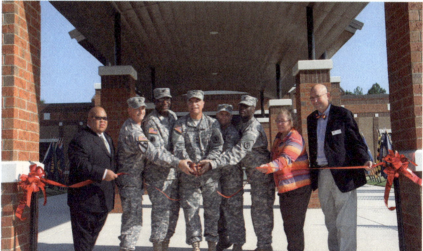

Figure 7-6. [Top] The ribbon cutting ceremony of the new blood donor center at Ft Bragg. Colonel Ronny Fryar is joined by senior officers from Womack Army Medical Center and Ft Bragg. Courtesy of the Ft Bragg Blood Donor Center.

Figure 7-7. [Bottom] The ribbon cutting ceremony of the new Sullivan Memorial Blood Center on Ft Benning. Colonel Frank Rentas and Major Matthew Swingholm participate. Courtesy of the Sullivan Memorial Blood Center, Ft Benning, Georgia.

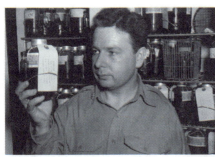

Figure 7-8. Lieutenant Colonel Eugene R. Sullivan, a physician who served during World War II and researched the use of blood in the treatment of the wounded. Courtesy of the Sullivan Memorial Blood Center, Ft Benning, Georgia.

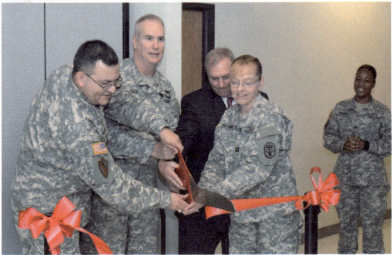

Figure 7-9. The ribbon cutting ceremony of the new Kendrick Memorial Blood Donor Center on June 12, 2014. Colonel Richard Gonzales is joined by Lieutenant Colonel (Ret) Kevin Belanger; Captain Wendy Adamian; and Colonel John Lamoureaux, Commander, Eisenhower Army Medical Center. Courtesy of the Kendrick Memorial Blood Center, Ft Gordon, Georgia.

contributed to the FDA approval of the first additive solution in 30 years. The new solution, AS-7 (SOLX: Hemerus Medical, LLC, St. Paul, MN), was approved by the FDA for a 42-day shelf life. This improved solution preserves the red cells much better than other similar solutions because it reduces cell aging, which normally occurs during storage.[11] He continued his work on the whole blood pathogen reduction device (WB PRD) and rapid transfusion transmitted disease detection (RT2D2) device, serving as program manager.

Research and development will remain important. The ABP continues to seek ways to reduce the risks associated with blood product transfusions and to find more effective and efficient ways of treating the wounded on the battlefield.

LOOKING FORWARD

As we look into the future for ways to improve hemorrhage control and fluid resuscitation as close to the point of injury as possible, we can reflect on the past. One past reflection consists of the efforts to develop a new generation of freeze-dried plasma. During World War II and the Korean War, freeze-dried plasma was used to provide a means of resuscitation far forward on the battlefield. Logistically, it was a better way to provide plasma compared to frozen or liquid plasma products. Unfortunately, many patients developed post-transfusion hepatitis, and the use of this product eventually ended. Colonel Gonzales' focus on battlefield requirements was also instrumental in ASBP's collaboration with the French military blood program to develop a new generation of a freeze-dried plasma product through an expanded access investigational new drug application overseen by both the FDA and the military institutional review board. This product will be used by US special operations forces. As part of the collaboration project, the ABP coordinates the collection of plasmapheresis units at donor centers and ships them to France, where they freeze-dry the plasma and return it to the United States. Once the FDA licenses the product, it will be available for use across the military.[12]

The French military has been using this freeze-dried plasma product for years, and it is registered and monitored by France's regulating agencies.[13] Unlike the past, modern era infectious disease testing is performed on the plasma. Donor pools are now much smaller, with fewer than 11 donors per pool compared to hundreds of donors per donor pool previously. The significantly reduced number of donors is attributed to the use of plasmapheresis units instead of whole blood–derived plasma. The freeze-dried plasma from this collaborative effort will meet the requirement as development and licensure efforts within the United States move forward.[14]

As once was done decades ago, having low titer, Group O whole blood available at the point of injury provides wounded soldiers a greater chance of survival. The initial effort was through a program known as Ranger Group O Low Titer (ROLO) Fresh Whole Blood Program. The concept was spearheaded by Lieutenant Colonel Andre Cap, chief of blood research at the Army Institute of Surgical Research and Lieutenant Colonel Jason Corley, deputy director of the Army Blood Program.[15] In May 2015, Lieutenant Colonel Melanie Sloan led the staff of the Sullivan Memorial Blood Center in a key role in establishing the program with the 75th Ranger Regiment.[16] The objective of the program is to prescreen soldiers to serve as donors should fresh whole blood be needed for the immediate treatment of the wounded.[16] In addition to standard donor testing, titers for anti-A and anti-B are also determined. If the titer is less that 1:256, it is considered low titer.[15] All results are entered into the Theater Medical Data Store for use by the regiment medical staff. Over the next year and a half, this program was expanded to all Ranger battalions and several Special Forces groups.[17] Nearly two years later, the Army Material Command recognized the Ranger Group O Low Titer (ROLO) Fresh Whole Blood Program as a winner of the Army's Greatest Innovation Award.[15]

In April 2016, a related effort began at the direction of the ASBPO. Each Service blood program was requested to begin producing low titer Group O whole blood. All of the Army blood donor center have been licensed by the FDA to produce whole blood, but none were producing a specific product to be distributed outside their facility. As of March 2017, the Army Blood Program had a requirement of 30 to 32 units of low titer Group O whole blood each week for US Central Command. Colonel Taylor predicts that this requirement will grow in the future especially if it is expanded to medical evacuation flights, and is kept as contingency inventory in support of rapid deploying units on Ft Bragg and Ft Campbell. She also noted that the San Antonio Military Medical Center plans to begin use of low titer Group O whole blood sometime in 2017 in support of their Level I trauma center.[18]

SUMMARY

The ABP has collected millions of units of blood to support US military members and beneficiaries in peacetime and war. The support of dedicated staff and generous donors within the military community made this possible. Many great leaders have continued to direct the program through countless changes and events. Our predecessors built a strong and successful program. Acknowledging that legacy, present leaders should be reminded of what Colonel Frank Camp noted, "We stand on the shoulders of giants."[19]

REFERENCES

1. US Army Blood Program. US Army Blood Program Strategic Plan 2012–2015. September 2011. Located at: US Army Medical Department Museum, San Antonio, TX.
2. US Department of the Army. Don't ask, don't tell. http://www.army.mil/dadt. Accessed August 23, 2013.
3. Headquarters, US Army Medical Command. *Implementation of the AABB Full-Length Donor History Questionnaire (DHQ) with Accompanying Materials, and Implementation of ABPSOP B.201, Donor Medical History – Allogeneic*. Fort Sam Houston, TX: Department of the Army; November 5, 2012. Policy letter 2012-11-02.
4. AABB (formerly known as the American Association of Blood Banks). *AABB Business Associate Agreement for Accredited Facilities*. Bethesda, MD: Army Blood Program Office; 2011.
5. Harmening DM. *Modern Blood Banking and Transfusion Practices*. Philadelphia, PA: FA Davis Company; 2012.

6. US Food and Drug Administration, Center for Biologics Evaluation and Research (CBER). *Final Guidance on the Use of Serological Tests to Reduce the Risk of Transmission of Trypanosoma cruzi Infection in Whole Blood and Blood Components Intended for Transfusion.* Rockville, MD: FDA; 2010.
7. Headquarters, US Army Medical Command. *Policy on Donor Screening, Deferral and Look Back for Trypanosoma cruzi Infection/Chagas Disease.* Fort Sam Houston, TX: Department of the Army; November 22, 2011. Policy letter 2011-11-02.
8. Stramer SL, Hollinger FB, Katz LM, et al. Emerging infectious disease agents and their potential threat to transfusion safety. *Transfusion.* 2009;49:1S–29S.
9. Longacre E. Blood center gets a new home. Armed Services Blood Program website. http://www.militaryblood.dod.mil/ViewContent.aspx?con_id_pk=1633&fr=s. Published June 18, 2014. Accessed June 26, 2014.
10. Kuczmanski LA. Fort Bliss opens doors to new donor center. Armed Services Blood Program website. http://www.militaryblood.dod.mil/ViewContent.aspx?con_id_pk=1887. Published June 10, 2015. Accessed June 23, 2017.
11. US Food and Drug Administration. SOLX® System. Vaccines, blood, & biologics web page. http://www.fda.gov/biologicsbloodvaccines/bloodbloodproducts/approvedproducts/newdrugapplicationsndas/ucm349798.htm. May 24, 2013 update. Accessed September 16, 2014.
12. News 4 San Antonio. Freeze-dried plasma saves special ops soldier. https://www.youtube.com/watch?v=ndpyAkYAt70&list=UUgi5HggiWdSvL6g9oy2H86w. Published August 1, 2014. Accessed April 25, 2017.
13. Sailliol S, Martinaud C, Cap AP, et al. The evolving role of lyophilized plasma in remote damage control resuscitation in the French Armed Forces Health Services. *Transfusion.* 2013;53(suppl 1):65S–71S.
14. Gonzales R, Taylor AL, Atkinson AJ, Malloy WW, Macdonald VW, Cap AP. US Army blood program: 2025 and beyond. *Transfusion.* 2016;56(suppl 1):S85–S93.
15. Mayne T. Ranger whole blood program wins an Army's greatest innovation award. US Army Official website. https://www.army.mil/article/184219/ranger_whole_blood_program_wins_an_armys_greatest_innovation_award. Published March 14, 2017. Accessed June 23, 2017.
16. Longacre E. Military blood program surges into the future. US Military Blood Program website. http://www.militaryblood.dod.mil/viewcontent.aspx?con_id_pk=2377. Published May 22, 2017. Accessed October 5, 2017.
17. US Army Blood Program. Advances in the use of whole blood in combat trauma resuscitation. Military Health System and the Defense Health Agency Website https://health.mil/Reference-Center/Presentations?query=advances+in+the+use+of+whole+blood+in+combat+trauma+resuscitation. Published June 2, 2016. Accessed October 5, 2017.
18. Taylor A. Army Blood Program update. Talk presented at: Clinical Laboratory Management Association KnowledgeLab2017; March 26, 2017; Nashville, TN.
19. Camp FR, Conte N, Brewer JR. *Military Blood Banking 1941–1973—Lessons Learned Applicable to Civil Disasters and Other Considerations.* Fort Knox, KY: US Army Medical Research Laboratory, Blood Bank Center; 1973.

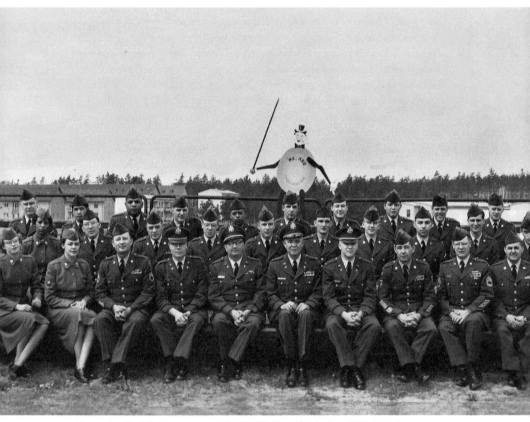

Figure 8-1. The US Army Europe (USAREUR) Blood Bank circa 1955. Captain Frank Camp is pictured in the front row, center. Courtesy of Colonel (Ret) Anthony Polk.

CHAPTER EIGHT

The Evolution of Army Blood Supply Units

The blood program of the US Army historically adapted to changes in requirements based on military strategy and operations. Organizational adaptability enabled the Army to use the most advanced technologies of the time to ensure that blood products were as safe and readily available as possible. Military units were developed and modified as needed over the years to address the need for blood collection and distribution in the continental United States and across the globe during peacetime and war. These units weathered changes in force structure and size, command reorganization and consolidation, and supply chain and management challenges. Through all these trials, the mission continued. The many lives saved are a testament to the effectiveness of the units that ensured blood products reached those in need.

BLOOD SUPPORT UNIT BEGINNINGS

Blood support units can trace their origins to World War II. Early in 1944, blood banks, or transfusion units, were established as part of deployed medical laboratories. Collection and transportation were their primary missions. As the war progressed, the Army established formal transfusion units. The 6713th Blood Transfusion Unit was the first numbered unit. This new unit was activated on May 9, 1944, and was attached to the 15th Medical General Laboratory, which provided additional personnel and testing when the requirement for blood increased. A few months later, the 6703rd Blood Transfusion Unit was activated. These units were organized with a base operation that focused on blood collections and forward distribution detachments.[1]

BLOOD UNITS SUPPORTING EUROPE

After World War II, blood bank detachments were deactivated or consolidated. In May 1949, the Army activated the 26th and 27th Blood Bank Bleeding Detachments. In May 1952 these two detachments were assigned to Landstuhl Army Medical Center in Germany with attachment to the 4th Medical Laboratory. At the same time, the 518th Blood Bank Detachment from Walter Reed General Hospital joined the other two detachments at Landstuhl. Two years later, in 1954, these three detachments were transferred to the 10th Medical Laboratory, where they remained until a reorganization and name change in 1960. In September of that year a new unit was activated, and on October 20 it was designated as the US Army Transfusion Service Unit, Europe. These MTOE (Modified Table of Organization and Equipment) units (26th, 27th, and 518th) were deactivated, and the new unit was designated as a TDA (Table of Distribution and Allowances) unit, without a combat role. One reference referred to this new unit as the 3741st US Army Transfusion Service Unit, Europe.[2] Normally TDA units were not designated with numerical identification. The new unit consisted of a headquarters, a processing and storage branch, a distribution section, and three collecting teams. A Medical Service Corps (MSC) officer led each of the collecting teams. Commanders of the US Army Transfusion Service Unit, Europe, included Major Claude Lenn, MSC; Lieutenant Colonel Michael Skvorak, MSC; and Lieutenant Colonel John Flintjer, MSC. The unit was more commonly known as the US Army Europe (USAREUR) Blood Bank (Figure 8-1), as certified by the AABB (formerly the American Association of Blood Banks). Its primary mission was to collect blood from US donors and supply the Army medical treatment centers throughout Europe. Each military hospital in Europe maintained a small donor center, usually for emergency collections. Training was another important mission. Once each month the USAREUR Blood Bank offered a weeklong training course on techniques in advanced blood banking. The class trained blood bank technicians on how to manage unusual and complex problems that might be encountered.[2–6]

Toward the end of 1966, the Army reorganized the USAREUR Blood Bank and gave it a new designation, the 655th Medical Company (Blood Bank). Its first commander was Major James E. Watt, MSC. When the last of the US forces left France as part of downsizing and restructuring, the overall layout of the forces stationed in Europe changed. During this time, the USAREUR surgeon considered reorganizing the medical structure and decided to create a new medical command to oversee Europe. On July 1, 1968, the US Army Medical Command Europe (USAMEDCOMEUR) was activated in Heidelberg, Germany. Initially the new command was subordinate to the Theater Army Support Command, but in 1973 USAMEDCOMEUR was realigned under USAREUR. The 655th

Medical Company (Blood Bank) was one of a handful of units assigned directly to USAMEDCOMEUR. It consisted of a headquarters (Team AJ), two blood processing detachments (Team NA), up to six blood collection detachments (Team NB), and six blood distribution detachments (Team NC).[7–9]

Early on, the 655th participated in Army training tests and operational readiness tests. The Army training test was a formal test with evaluators assigned from USAMEDCOMEUR that scrutinized all aspects of the unit from vehicles, to barracks, to unit funds, to weapons, and all types of maintenance. Problems of support from other commands or operational problems of any general or specific nature could be discussed. Aggressor forces were assigned to test the unit's defensive capability. The 655th was then tested to determine whether it could collect and process blood at sites other than the home station at Landstuhl. Operational readiness tests, however, were a little less formal. One operational readiness test was conducted in January 1970 at the unit's emergency site, a minimally heated warehouse in Baumholder, Germany. The blood bank center at Ft Knox shipped several hundred donor samples for processing and comparison with Ft Knox results. The ABO blood group results were fine, but the Rh results did not match well. On investigation, Captain Tobias realized that the Rh typing sera were manufactured for use at 70°F (21°C), and not at 50°F (10°C). During a winter Army training test, the 655th attempted to establish the NA team (blood processing) under canvas instead of using the warehouse. One day during the exercise, a moderate soaking rain in Baumholder threatened to turn to snow. Unloading heavy MTOE equipment, such as the floor-model specimen centrifuges, from the 2½-ton trucks and then carrying it over the mud into general purpose medium tents was daunting. When the 5-kW generators were started, power cables were lying in mud puddles, and Captain Tobias terminated that portion of the exercise. He initiated a change in the MTOE to add expandable vans for the NA team as well as equipment to better communicate with air ambulances. During another winter Army training test, the rain turned to snow, and 4 to 6 inches accumulated. When driving up a long 30-degree incline leading away from Baumholder, the team lost two 2½-ton trucks and a ¾-ton truck after they slid off the road. Luckily, no personnel suffered significant injuries, according to Kenneth Tobias' email dated October 2014.

One of the early real-world scenarios to affect the 655th Medical Company occurred in September 1970. Tensions between Palestinians and Jordanians erupted into civil war over control of Jordan. With the possibility of the United States and the Soviet Union entering the conflict, Captain Tobias, the commander of the 655th, received a call to ship all units of blood on hand to assets that the Department of Defense had deployed as a forward presence. USAMEDCOMEUR directed the 655th to collect as much blood as possible.

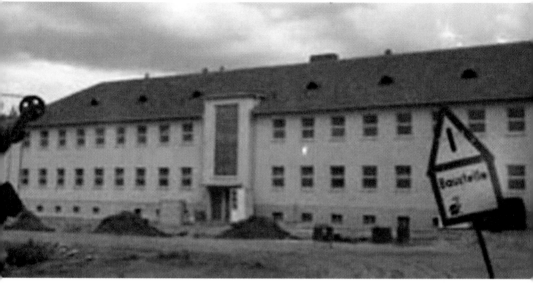

Figure 8-2. The old 10th Medical Laboratory building at Landstuhl, Germany, that was shared with the 655th Medical Company (Blood Bank). Courtesy of Armed Services Blood Program Office.

With the two NB teams (blood collecting) at full strength, the 655th could collect 400 units per day on a sustained basis. To collect more would require activating the four remaining NB teams and two additional NC teams (blood distribution). Captain Tobias quickly saw that it would not be easy to find enough donors to meet the requirement of 400 units per day. With the current collecting and processing tasks, donor recruitment was difficult. USAMEDCOMEUR tasked the commanders of the 2nd General Hospital and the 10th Medical Laboratory to conduct donor recruitment. US military units were placed on alert, but ultimately did not become directly involved in the conflict, according to Kenneth Tobias' email dated October 2014.

As the years passed, the mission of the US forces in Europe persisted. On September 21, 1978, the 7th Medical Command was activated, replacing USARMEDCOMEUR, which had no combat role. In November 1978 the 10th Medical Laboratory assumed operational control of the 655th Medical Company (Figures 8-2 to 8-4), although the 655th commander reported to the chief of professional services at the 7th Medical Command in Heidelburg, Germany (Attachment 8-1). The unit routinely participated in the major theater exercise, REFORGER (Return of Forces to Germany), and it was commanded by many Army blood bank officers. Following Major Watt were Captain Kenneth Tobias,[10] Lieutenant Colonel Joseph Tuggle (Figure 8-5) (BBF class of '62–63), Lieutenant

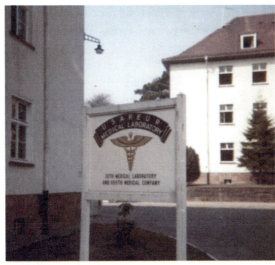

Figure 8-3. [Top] Billets of the 655th Medical Company (Blood Bank) circa 1972. Courtesy of Colin Michaud, assigned to the 655th Medical Company (Blood Bank) from January 1972 to May 1974.

Figure 8-4. [Bottom] The 655th Medical Company (Blood Bank) motor pool. Courtesy of Colin Michaud, assigned to the 655th from January 1972 to May 1974.

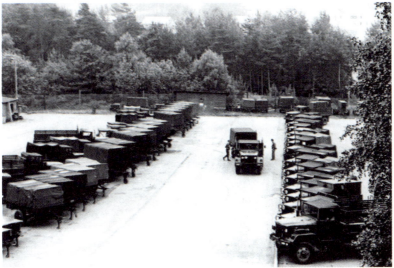

Colonel William Collins,[11] Lieutenant Colonel Jerry Brewer, Major Tony Polk, Major Tom Hathaway (BBF class of '80–81), Major Larry Feltz (BBF class of '77–78), Major Richard Brown, Major Mike Stanton, Lieutenant Colonel Wilbur Malloy, Major Robert Borowski, and Lieutenant Colonel John Hatten (BBF class of '82–83).

The 655th was FDA licensed and conducted blood drives throughout Germany for many years. A popular blood drive was held annually in Berlin and also in military communities in West Germany, according to Colonel (Retired)

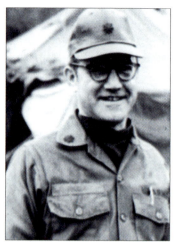

Figure 8-5. Lieutenant Colonel Joseph Tuggle. Commander, 655th Medical Company (Blood Bank) circa 1972. Courtesy of Colin Michaud, assigned to the 655th from January 1972 to May 1974.

Anthony Polk's email dated March 2014 and Colonel (Retired) Richard Brown's email dated June 2014.

The 655th was computerized around 1986 with a Kontron Automation system (Kontron; Augsberg, Germany) that Major Feltz ordered before he relinquished command. Major Stanton was the project officer when the system arrived. Colonel Richard Brown (Figure 8-6) and Major Mike Stanton initiated human immunodeficiency virus (HIV) and hepatitis C testing in theater for the blood supply, according to Colonel (Retired) Richard Brown's email dated August 2014.

BLOOD UNITS SUPPORTING KOREA

Early in 1980, Colonel James Spiker (Figure 8-7) summoned Captain Richard Platte, a newly assigned clinical laboratory officer for the 121st Evacuation Hospital and US Army Hospital in Seoul, to OTSG for a briefing on the current state of the Korea area blood program. The program had atrophied over the years, and Colonel Spiker directed Captain Platte to revitalize it immediately upon his arrival in March 1980. Like previous laboratory officers, Captain Platte was also the Korea area blood program officer. He began making significant changes and improvements to the blood teams that were attached to US Army Medical Command, Korea. With the help of the commander, Colonel Lewis Mologne;

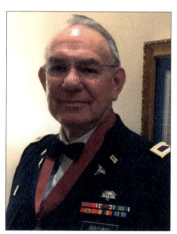

Figure 8-6. Colonel Richard Brown. Courtesy of Colonel (Ret) Richard Brown.

the US Army Community Hospital, Seoul; and the 121st Evacuation Hospital, Captain Platte corrected the teams' readiness deficiencies, according to Colonel (Retired) Richard Platte's email dated June 2014. Colonel Mologne was an ideal leader to advise and assist blood team operational improvements since he wore several hats and had broad perspective and experience. He was simultaneously commander of US Army Medical Command, Korea; the surgeon of United Nations Command/US Forces Korea/Eighth US Army; and the commander of the 121st Evacuation Hospital in Seoul, Korea.

Following Captain Platte in 1982, Captain Wilbur Malloy continued his predecessor's work, making improvements in the blood bank operations. He also worked on war plans, exercise plans, and improved the theater's blood program regulation. Malloy and the blood bank teams participated in numerous exercises, including Team Spirit and Ulchi Focus Lens. He demonstrated the capability of delivering large quantities of blood products using the low-altitude parachute extraction procedure in Osan, Korea (Figures 8-8 and 8-9), and the Naval Emergency Cargo Air Delivery Systems in the Sea of Japan. Both operations were successful and confirmed that large palletized quantities of blood could be delivered by the two parachute procedures, according to Colonel (Retired) Anthony Polk's email dated June 2014. This operational structure of the theater blood program continued until 1987.

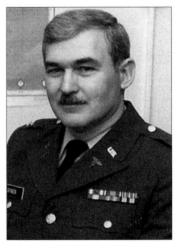

Figure 8-7. Colonel James Spiker Jr. Courtesy of Colonel (Ret) James Spiker Jr.

Seeing a need to establish a formal military structure to manage the theater blood program on the peninsula, the Army decided that a unit like the 655th was needed in Korea. The 461st Medical Company (Blood Bank) was activated early in 1987 in Yongsan, Korea, attached to the 18th Medical Command. Major Bruce Sylvia was the first blood bank officer to command the 461st. The 461st commander also assumed the responsibilities of the Korea Area Joint Blood Program, which was responsible for Army, Navy, and Air Force blood requirements on the Korean peninsula, according to Colonel (Retired) Bruce Sylvia's email dated June 2014. In the summer of 1989, Major Noel Webster (Figure 8-10) (BBF class of '88–89) assumed command of the 461st. He began working with the US Army's Health Facilities Planning Agency to gain approval for and design the frozen blood depots at Camp Carroll and Camp Humphreys, helping to meet Military Blood Program 2004's objective for the use of frozen blood. Major Webster also set up blood donor enzyme immunoassay testing on the Abbott system at Supply Point 51 in Yongson. Other blood bank officers, including Major Gary Norris and Major Elaine Perry, commanded the 461st as well, according to Colonel (Retired) Steve Beardsley's email dated February 2014.

Figure 8-8. [Top] A Container Delivery Drop during a field exercise in Korea. Courtesy of the Armed Services Blood Program Office.

Figure 8-9. [Bottom Left] A Container Delivery Drop during a field exercise in Korea (on the ground). Courtesy of the Armed Services Blood Program Office.

Figure 8-10. [Bottom Right] Major Noel Webster examines two "training units" during a field exercise in Korea. Courtesy of Kathleen Elder.

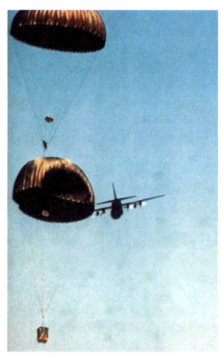

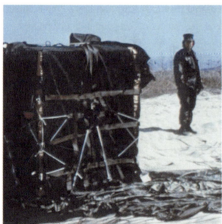

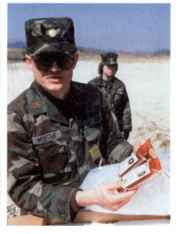

As part of the Medical Force 2000 reorganization efforts, Major Don Fipps (BBF class of '87–88) developed a new blood supply unit to replace the medical company (blood bank), according to Colonel (Retired) Richard Brown's email dated June 2014. These new Medical Force 2000 blood bank platoons were activated under the redesigned medical logistics battalions. The blood bank platoons consisted of 20 personnel assigned to a headquarters, a storage and distribution squad to manage 3,000 units per day, and a processing squad that focused on frozen red cells that had been prepositioned in a theater when directed.

Prior to this, blood was managed separately. During the post–Operation Desert Storm drawdown and Medical Force 2000 restructuring, blood was managed with all Class VIII (medical) supplies. This and the fact that the platoons were attached to medical logistics battalions helped streamline operations and improve blood support in theaters.

In the spring of 1994, after a short 7 years, the 461st was deactivated and replaced by the blood bank platoon under the 16th Medical Logistics Battalion. Shortly after that, the 655th was replaced by the blood bank platoon underneath the 226th Medical Logistics Battalion in October 1994, according to Colonel (Retired) Steve Beardsley's email dated February 2014.

MEDICAL REENGINEERING AND BLOOD UNITS

In 2002, in accordance with the Medical Reengineering Initiative, the Medical Force 2000 blood bank platoons were replaced with blood support detachments (BSDs) attached to medical logistics battalion. BSDs consisted of 30 personnel divided into three sections: (1) a headquarters, (2) collection and manufacturing, and (3) storage and distribution. A BSD could collect up to 432 donations, produce 432 units of packed red blood cells, and distribute 33 boxes (when not collecting or manufacturing) every day. The detachment also stored up to 4,080 units of red blood cells.[12] The unit conversion took a few years, but eventually five BSDs were activated:

(1) 153rd BSD at Ft Lewis
(2) 440th BSD at Ft Sam Houston
(3) 932nd BSD at Ft Hood
(4) 432nd BSD at Ft Bragg
(5) 95th BSD in Korea

Table 8-1 identifies the commanders of these five BSDs from activation date to the present.

As the wars in Afghanistan and Iraq continued, it soon became evident that the current configuration of the BSD was too large and lacked the flexibility to best support the theater of operation. After many years of work by the Army Medical Department's Forces Design Update, the BSD was reconfigured into the medical detachment, blood support (MDBS) beginning late in 2011. While at the Directorate of Combat and Doctrine Development, Colonel Richard Gonzales (BBF class of '92–93) focused on the final stages of the redesign. The five active component units remained, and the reserve component gained two detachments. All MDBSs now fell under the command and control of the Headquarters,

Headquarters Detachment, multifunctional medical battalion. The new design increased mobility and modularity and facilitated the ability to conduct split operations more effectively than the previous BSD design. The MDBS consists of a headquarters and three teams: (1) a collection, storage, and distribution team; (2) a collection, manufacturing, and distribution team; and (3) a distribution team.[12] Storage capacity is up to 5,100 units of blood.[13] Additional changes included a reduction of personnel from 30 to 22, the addition of plateletpheresis, and the removal of frozen red cell storage and deglycerolization because the large freezers needed for these processes proved to be too heavy to move, according to Colonel Richard Gonzales' email dated May 2010. In fiscal year 2015, the MTOE was reduced by one medical laboratory specialist, bringing the total personnel to 21, according to Major Gerald Kellar's email dated August 2014. As the Army continues to change to meet the threats around the globe, changes in the blood support units are likely to occur to meet the ever-changing needs for blood support in military operations.

A NEW ENVIRONMENT

In September 2014, US Africa Command led an effort to provide logistical and engineering support to the West African countries of Guinea, Sierra Leone, and Liberia in response to the largest Ebola virus disease outbreak in history. The 440th Medical Detachment, Blood Support was called upon to play a role in this unique mission named Operation United Assistance. Major Matthew Swingholm, Joint Blood Program Officer for US European Command and US Africa Command, coordinated blood support in the region. Coordination among the 440th in Liberia, a Damage Control Resuscitation/Surgery Team, and the Monrovia Medical Unit facilitated full blood support capabilities.[14] The Monrovia Medical Unit was a unique 25 bed facility run by the US Public Health Commissioned Service and designed to care for workers who might become infected with Ebola while working with infected patients.[15] In addition to providing blood support, the soldiers of the 440th conducted plateletpheresis and emergency whole blood collection training; prescreened potential donors, creating a walking blood bank; and helped establish a self-sustaining blood program for the Monrovia Medical Unit.[14]

SUMMARY

Through the 20th century and into the 21st, the Army continually adjusted its strategy to meet the challenges of the time. So have the blood supply units of the Army. The changes have been in size, flexibility, and in the technology the units use. This evolution supported the goal of getting blood as far forward as possible, closest to the point of injury. Blood is a unique medical supply. Because it

Table 8-1. Commanders of blood support detachments/medical detachment, blood support

Unit	Activated	Commanders	Tenure
440th–Ft Sam Houston/Ft Bliss 440th BSD (Provisional)	Established January 17, 2002, activated June 16, 2002*	1LT Pablo Rivera	January 2002–February 2002
		MAJ David Reiber	February 2002–January 2004
		MAJ Kevin Belanger	January 2004–January 2006
		MAJ Matthew Swingholm	January 2006–July 2009
		CPT Craig Mester	July 2009–June 2011
		MAJ Jose Quesada	June 2011–September 2013
		1LT Hiram Virchis‡	September 2013–May 2014
		CPT Steven McDaniel	May 2014–July 2016
		MAJ Elaine Morrison	July 2016–Present
432nd–Ft Bragg	September 16, 2006	MAJ Audra Taylor	September 2006–July 2008
		MAJ Jason Corley	July 2008–May 2010
		MAJ Aleskey Cascofigeroa	May 2010–May 2012
		MAJ Javier Trevino	May 2012–March 2015
		MAJ Veronica Ortiz	March 2015–February 2017
		CPT William Ceballos	February 2017–Present
95th–Korea	April 14, 2005	2LT Luis Tejada	October 2008–November 2008
		CPT April Harris	November 2008–January 2011
		CPT Semone Dilworth	January 2011–January 2014
		CPT Chih Huang	January 2014–February 2016
		CPT Vincent Duncan	February 2016–March 2017
		CPT Manuela Bauldy	March 2017–Present

Table 8-1. Commanders of blood support detachments/medical detachment, blood support (continued)

Unit	Activated	Commanders	Tenure
932nd–Ft Hood	April 14, 2005	MAJ Barbara Bachman	April 2005–July 2008
		MAJ Teresa Terry	July 2008–January 2011
		MAJ Harry McDonald Jr	January 2011–December 2012
		CPT Jack Alley (HHC)†	December 2012–January 2013
		1LT Nathan Baker†	January 2013–February 2013
		CPT Ronnie Hill	February 2013–July 2015
		CPT Joseph Cheser	July 2015–May 2017
		CPT Joshua Kuper	May 2017–Present
153rd–Ft Lewis	September 16, 2006	MAJ Melanie Sloan	September 2006–January 2009
		MAJ Christopher Evans	January 2009–March 2012
		MAJ Gerald Kellar	March 2012–December 2013
		MAJ Jocelyn Advlento	December 2013–November 2014
		CPT Jacquelyn Messenger	November 2014–May 2016
		MAJ Juan Guzman	May 2016–Present

BSD: Blood Support Detachment; 1LT: First Lieutenant; MAJ: Major; 2LT: Second Lieutenant; CPT: Captain; HHC: Headquarters and Headquarters Company

* The 440th was a provisional unit for 6 months prior to its formal activation date. First Lieutenant Rivera was commander while the unit was in garrison. The provisional unit deployed in January 2002. On November 13, 2013, the 440th completed rebasing operations at Ft Sam Houston and reorganized at Ft Bliss as a direct reporting unit to the 31st Combat Support Hospital.
† Acting commander

Data source: Army Blood Program Office.

is a living, biological product, it is distinctly different than other medical supplies. Officers and noncommissioned officers specifically trained in collecting, managing, and distributing blood products are the reason for the success of the blood supply units. By providing the right blood products, in the right amount, at the right time, these units have created a successful legacy of saving lives on the battlefield.

REFERENCES

1. Kendrick DB. *Blood Program in World War II*. Washington, DC: Department of the Army; 1964.
2. US Army Transfusion Unit, Europe. *Med Bull US Army Europe*. 1964;21(4):119–121. http://stimson.contentdm.oclc.org/cdm/singleitem/collection/p15290coll5/id/1797/rec/1. Accessed September 2, 2014.
3. US Army Transfusion Service Unit, Europe *Med Bull US Army Europe*. 1962;19:255–257. http://stimson.contentdm.oclc.org/cdm/singleitem/collection/p15290coll5/id/4035/rec/3. Accessed September 2, 2014.
4. Notes from the Office of the Surgeon. *Med Bull US Army Europe*. 1963;20:3–8. http://stimson.contentdm.oclc.org/cdm/singleitem/collection/p15290coll5/id/3983/rec/12. Accessed September 2, 2014.
5. USAREUR Medical Laboratory. *Med Bull US Army Europe*. 1961;18:172–175,180. http://stimson.contentdm.oclc.org/cdm/singleitem/collection/p15290coll5/id/3966/rec/1. Accessed September 2, 2014.
6. Bosman RI. Blood –the two-edged sword. *Med Bull US Army Europe*. 1967;24:6–7. http://stimson.contentdm.oclc.org/cdm/singleitem/collection /p15290coll5/id/2452/rec/8. Accessed September 2, 2014.
7. Medical memos. *Med Bull US Army Europe*. 1978;35. http://stimson.contentdm.oclc.org/cdm/singleitem/collection/p15290coll5/id/1379/rec/1. Accessed September 2, 2014.
8. Medical memos. *Med Bull US Army Europe*. 1973;30. http://stimson.contentdm.oclc.org/cdm/singleitem/collection/p15290coll5/id/1455/rec/1. Accessed: September 2, 2014.
9. US Department of the Army. *Medical Support Theater of Operations*. Washington, DC: DA; April 1970: Chap 8. Field Manual 8-10.
10. Camp FR Jr, Conte NF, German NI, Nalbandian RM, Kaplan HS, Tobias KI. Progress notes in military blood banking: a systematic approach to early recognition and treatment of incompatible blood transfusion injury. *Med Bull US Army Europe*. 1972;67–75. http://cdm15290.contentdm.oclc.org/cdm/ref/collection/p15290coll5/id/2650. Accessed September 25, 2014.
11. Blood is good as gold but not so durable. *Stars and Stripes* [European edition]. December 31, 1974:9.

12. Gonzales R. Army combat developments and the laboratory. Paper presented at: Society of Armed Forces Medical Laboratory Scientists (SAFMLS) 2010 Annual Meeting; March 24, 2010; San Diego, CA. http://www.safmls.org/2010/2010_annual_meeting_presentations.html. Published March 24, 2010. Updated May 23, 2013. Accessed May 25, 2017.
13. US Department of the Army. *Army Health System*. Washington, DC: DA; August 2013. Field Manual 4-02.
14. Terry T. 440th BSD supports Operation United Assistance. Armed Services Blood Program website. http://www.militaryblood.dod.mil/ViewContent.aspx?con_id_pk=1779&fr=s&i=l. Published January 2, 2015. Accessed June 23, 2017.
15. Hoskins N. Ebola treatment unit for medical workers to open. US Army Official website. https://www.army.mil/article/137701/Ebola_treatment_unit_for_medical_workers_to_open/. Published November 6, 2014. Accessed June 23, 2017.

DEPARTMENT OF THE ARMY
HEADQUARTERS, 10TH MEDICAL LABORATORY
APO NEW YORK 09180

AEMML-CO   1 November 1978

MEMORANDUM FOR CDR, 655TH MEDICAL COMPANY

SUBJECT: Relationship of 10th Medical Laboratory and 655th Medical Company (Blood Bank)

1. Per instructions received from Executive Officer 7th Medical Command dated 16 October 1978, OPCON of the 655th Medical Company (Blood Bank) passes to the 10th Medical Laboratory. The message states that appropriate changes to 7th Medical Command Regulation 10-5 are to be forthcoming.

2. In order to provide interim guidance relating to this change in management structure, written (interim) statements of operational principles, goals, and specific tasking assignments are felt to be appropriate. Until further guidance is received, Memoranda such as these will serve as the source of guidance for operation of the 655th Medical Company (Blood Bank).

3. Status of Commander, 655th Medical Company: It is assumed that the 655th Medical Company will continue as a separately identified unit (to provide maximum flexibility in war-time situations), therefore, the duties of the Commander 655th Medical Company are not expected to be greatly altered except that operational objectives and specific mission related instructions, as necessary, will be issued by the Commander, 10th Medical Laboratory.

4. Efficiency Reports: The subject of how efficiency reports are to be ultimately handled is to be determined by the 7th Medical Command. It is reasonable to assume that the Commander, 10th Medical Laboratory will rate the Commander, 655th Medical Company and that further considerations of the rating scheme will follow as determined by appropriate headquarters. No action, however, will be taken until further guidance in this matter is received.

5. 10th Medical Laboratory Support: In order to provide optimum support without losing the capabilities of the 655th Medical Company to operate independently in wartime, the medical laboratory supply and administrative services will assist and strengthen, but not replace

Attachment 8-1.

AEMML-CO
MEMORANDUM FOR CDR, 655TH MEDICAL COMPANY
1 November 1978

present 655th Medical Company self support activities. The Executive Officer, 10th Medical Laboratory, will issue a separate (temporary) Memorandum concerning this subject. Where the 655th Medical Company has a requirement for support and lacks organic capability (such as the use of a Language Translator) the 10th Medical Laboratory will provide such services if such internal capability exists.

6. Principles of Operations: Present day principles governing operations of American blood banks must be complied with during peace time operations. In line with the present operational structure of blood banks in CONUS, the following guidlines are appropriate.

   a. The "prototype" community blood bank operation in America has a Board of Governors composed of members of medical community activities as its final authority. Serving under the Board of Governors are (generally) these individuals with clearly defined areas of responsibility.

      (1) The medical director

      (2) The technical director

      (3) The administrator

It is desirable that peace time blood bank operations for the US Army in Europe should follow functional organizational policies as follows:

      (1) 7th Medical Command is the military equivalent of the civilian "Board of Directors".

      (2) The Commander, 10th Medical Laboratory (or a fully qualified clinical pathologist appointed by the Commander, 10th Medical Laboratory) should act as "Medical Director".

      (3) The Commander, 655th Medical Company should act as "Technical Director" and "Chief Administrative Officer".

      (4) Where appropriate, inspection and accreditation by recognized professional associations should be sought.

7. War Missions:

   a. Possible wartime task for the blood bank require a large increase in blood bank capabilities. In addition, the 10th Medical Laboratory might be required to deploy one or more mobile laboratories

Attachment 8-1. Continued

AEMML-CO 1 November 1978
MEMORANDUM FOR CDR, 655TH MEDICAL COMPANY

with blood banking capabilities. This indicates a need for considerable cross training; such a program of "exchange" of laboratory technicians between the 10th Medical Laboratory and the 655th Medical Company will set up to start 20 November. At least two technicians will be on exchange rotation between the units at all times, until further notice.

    b. In order to stockpile some reserve of fresh frozen plasma, the 655th Medical Company will gradually embark on a program of providing only part of its RBC containing products as whole blood -- the rest will be packed cells (the percentage of packed cells to whole blood to increase as acceptance of the practice is gained at the hospitals served). This plasma will be processed and stored as fresh frozen for possible "war-reserve" use.

8. Equipment Plans (MEDCASE): Review and approval of eminent equipment purchases and future purchase plans is an appropriate function of a blood bank medical director. The Commander, 10th Medical Laboratory will perform this function for the 655th Medical Company. The 655th Medical Company will prepare a list of the status of current and planned MEDCASE acquisitions for such review.

9. Attendance of "Officers Call" and "Managers Meeting" of the 10th Medical Laboratories: The Commander, 655th Medical Company -- or, in his absence, an appropriate substitute, will attend Managers conferences. Officers of the 655th Medical Company are encouraged to attend 10th Medical Laboratory "Officers Call".

RICHARD H. STIENMIER
Colonel, MC
Commanding

CF:
CofS, 7th Medical Command
ACofS, Professional Service, Medical Command
Consultant in Surgery, Medical Command
Sub-community Commander, Landstuhl

Attachment 8-1. Continued

Final Thoughts

As the official blood program of the US military, the Armed Services Blood Program relies on coordination from the blood programs of each of the military services it represents—Army, Navy, and Air Force—as well as the unified and combatant commands. As a result, several components are always working together to provide quality blood products to ill or injured service members, retirees, and their families worldwide. The individual service blood program offices manage their respective blood programs and Food and Drug Administration licenses. While the Armed Services Blood Program has a long-standing history of its own, the individual blood programs for each service also carry a rich history of important events, regulations, and people that shaped the way they collect, manufacture, test, store, and ship blood products around the world. Along with our sister services, the Army Blood Program continues to grow and change as we strive towards meeting the requirements in an ever-changing world, from the battlefield to our superior healthcare system.

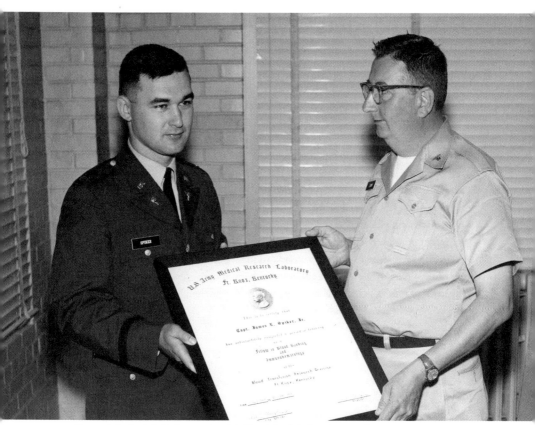

Figure A-2. Captain Spiker receives his Blood Bank Fellowship certificate from Lieutenant Colonel Frank Camp at the US Army Medical research Laboratory, Ft Knox, Kentucky, in 1966. Courtesy of Colonel (Ret) James Spiker Jr.

APPENDIX A
Army Blood Bank Fellowship

To meet military hospital and combat needs, the military requires qualified personnel to preserve a safe and secure blood supply. The US Army Blood Bank Fellowship (BBF) (Figure A-1) is an 18-month program that trains clinical laboratory officers from all three branches of the armed forces (Army, Navy, and Air Force) in the advanced and specialized blood bank topics required in today's healthcare industry. After completing the 18-month program (Figure A-2), officers graduate with a Master of Science degree from George Washington University. Students take courses in immunology, cellular and molecular biology, transfusion-transmitted diseases, transfusion services, and donor center operations and management. Other courses include accreditation and federal regulatory requirements, such as quality systems and current good manufacturing practices as established by the Food and Drug Administration and the AABB.

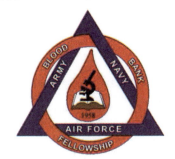

Figure A-1. The Blood Bank Fellowship (BBF) logo. Courtesy of Mr. Bill Turcan, US Army Blood Bank Fellowship.

The Commission on Accreditation of Allied Health Education Programs accredits the BBF, and the AABB sponsors the committee that conducts the accreditation process. The program consistently ranks in the top five of the 17 blood banking specialist programs in the United States. Currently, the BBF has a graduation rate nearing 98%—8% higher than the national average. The specialist in blood banking exam pass rate is around 90%—nearly double the national average.

The US Army BBF program was established in 1958 at Walter Reed Army Institute of Research in Washington, DC, by Colonel William H. Crosby, Medical Corps, chief of hematology, and Lieutenant Colonel Joseph H. Akeroyd, Medical Service Corps. The program's intent was to provide military officers with the

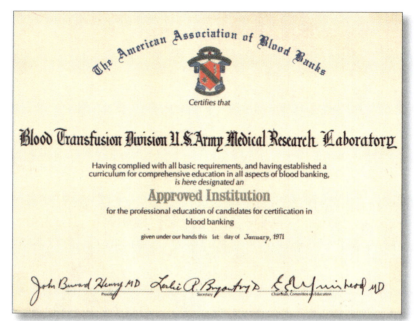

Exhibit A-1. Certification of Blood Transfusion Division U.S. Army Medical research Laboratory, Ft Knox, Kentucky, as an approved institute by the American Association of Blood Banks. January 1, 1971. Certificate from Camp Memorial Blood Center closure files. Courtesy of the Army Blood Program office.

training and experience to become experts and leaders in military blood banking in both peacetime and wartime. It was formally sponsored by the US Army and had academic affiliations with the US Navy and US Air Force through interservice memoranda of understanding. First Lieutenant William S. Collins II, US Army, was the first fellow.[1]

Colonel Crosby and Major Frank Camp, Medical Service Corps, established the blood research division in the US Army Medical Research Laboratory at Ft Knox, Kentucky, in 1965, and the BBF was transferred there. With the fellowship's relocation, the number of its allotted slots for Army officers increased from one to three.[2] The AABB designated the blood transfusion division as an "approved institution" for the professional education of candidates for certification in blood banking on January 1, 1971 (Exhibit A-1).

The DoD officially mandated the BBF in 1972. With the help of Dr. William Hann, a colonel in the US Army Reserve and professor of science at Bowling Green State University, Ohio, the BBF established an affiliation with the university in 1973 (Exhibit A-2). They gave academic credit for all clinical rotations and classroom lectures that the fellows participated in while at Walter Reed Army Medical Center. With additional graduate classes and successful completion of a thesis, the university granted Master of Science and Specialist in Applied Biology degrees to fellows who completed the program. The full degree program included 12 months for the initial specialist in blood banking portion and an additional 6 months for the master's degree. To consolidate resources, the program moved to the Blood Bank Center, also located at Ft Knox, in 1974. It remained at this location for another 2 years, until a Base Realignment and Closure Commission decision moved the program back to Walter Reed Army Medical Center in 1976.

In the late 1980s, an effort arose to remove the BBF from the Army sponsorship and transfer it to the Navy, for two main reasons. One reason was its affiliation with Bowling Green State University, which awarded graduate degrees at the completion of the fellowship. The second was that the program director of the fellowship, Lieutenant Colonel Richard Platte, did not have a PhD, while the Navy did have a blood officer with a PhD. Generally, graduate programs are headed by individuals who have earned doctorate degrees in their respective areas of expertise. Lieutenant Colonel Platte worked with Colonel James Spiker to designate the program director position as one of the validated positions requiring a PhD, to cement academic standing of the BBF. This was the first and only blood bank officer position on any TDA (Table of Distribution and Allowances) in the Army to also require a PhD. The first officer with a PhD assigned to this new position was Lieutenant Colonel Tom Hathaway (BBF class of '80–81), according to Colonel (Retired) Richard Platte's email dated November 2011.

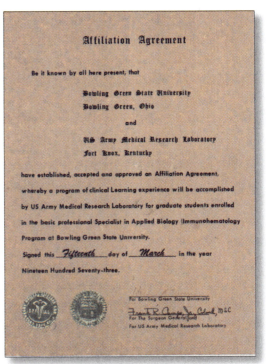

Exhibit A-2. Affiliation Agreement between Bowling Green State University and the US Army Medical Research Laboratory, Ft Knox, Kentucky. March 15, 1973. Document from the Camp Memorial Blood Center closure files. Courtesy of the Army Blood Program office.

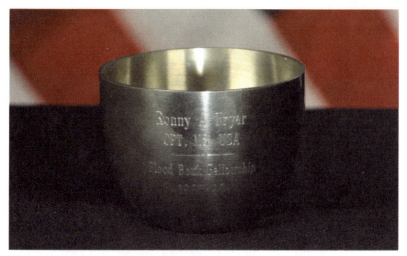

Figure A-3. The presentation of the Jefferson Cup is a long-held tradition. The cup is a symbol of academia to the Blood Bank Fellowship (BBF) graduates. The cup represents the history of the Armed Services Blood Program being passed to its future. BBF alumni purchase the cups for the graduating class. A Fellow is not allowed to drink anything from the cup until passing the Specialist in Blood Banking registry exam through the American Society of Clinical Pathologists. Courtesy of Colonel (Ret) Ronny Fryar.

As the director of the Army Blood Program, Colonel Richard Brown served on the advisory board for the BBF. He worked with the Walter Reed Army Medical Center directors of laboratory education and training, Lieutenant Colonel Mike Fitzpatrick and Lieutenant Colonel Mike Stanton, to change the fellowship's university affiliation because of costs and insufficient university involvement with the program, according to Colonel (Retired) Richard Brown's email dated September 2014. The BBF changed its affiliation to the George Washington University in 2000 because of these four factors:

1. Bowling Green State University charged the fellows out-of-state tuition.
2. Bowling Green State University charged for all program credits, even though it did not teach any of the fellowship courses.
3. George Washington University would only charge for the coursework it would teach.
4. As George Washington University moved more courses online, tuition costs decreased another 30%.

Although George Washington University is a private school with a higher tuition, the total costs to the fellows was about the same, but the university was now more involved with the students.

Table A-1. Graduates of the Blood Bank Fellowship

Walter Reed Institute of Research, Washington, DC		
Year	Graduates	Service
1958–1959	W.S. Collins	US Army
1959–1960	E.B. McCord	US Army
1960–1961	F.R. Camp	US Army
	R.N. Huff	US Air Force
1961–1962	A.M. Gottleib	US Army
1962–1963	J.M. Tuggle	US Army
1963–1964	T.F. Allen	US Army

US Army Medical Research Laboratory, Fort Knox, KY		
Year	Graduates	Service
1965–1966	J.R. Brewer, J.F. Rodgers, J.E. Spiker	US Army
1966–1967	D.G. Courtenay, G. Ikeda, M.H. McClain	US Army
1967–1968	S.S. Gates, H.C. Harrell, G.N. Sesano	US Army
1968–1969	J.D. Arnoldin, R.L. Phillips, J.H. Radcliffe	US Army
1969–1970	V.R. Coley, D.E. Hohn, B.J. Johnson	US Army
	D. Levan	US Navy
1970–1971	J.B. Beene	US Navy
	T.R. Lesser, B.Y. Linkenhoker, V.J. Simon	US Army
1971–1972	A.G. Cumze	US Air Force
	R.G. DeBonneville, L.R. McKinley, J.H. Young	US Army
	J.R. Maples	US Navy
1972–1973	S.S. Hill, S.A. Lavoy	US Air Force
	W.P. Monoghan	US Navy
	A.J. Polk, P.S. Sepulveda, D.E. Urban, R.T. Usry	US Army
	R.J. Tjan	Civilian
1973–1974	J.W. Bell, E.M. Frohman, W.E. Opie, R.L. Travis	US Army
	G.R. Koehn	US Navy
	C.A. Newberth-Bue	Civilian
	H.F. Wren	US Air Force

Table A-1. Graduates of the Blood Bank Fellowship, continued

The Blood Bank Center, Fort Knox, KY		
Year	Graduates	Service
1974–1975	F.M. Hack, K.A. Fontecchio, L.E. Lippert, A.B. Papineau	US Army
	B.J. Sawyer	US Air Force
1975–1976	R.E. Duhon	US Air Force
	S.E. Knodel, K.E. Zielmanski	US Army

Walter Reed Army Medical Center, Washington, DC		
Year	Graduates	Service
1976–1977	B.F. Chaney, W.W. Malloy	US Army
	J.R. Lindberg	US Navy
	R.C. Vura	US Air Force
1977–1978	L.C. Feltz, R.G. Sullivan	US Army
	D.A. Reichman	US Navy
1978–1979	D.A. Smith, T.S. Wadsworth	US Navy
1979–1980	D.A. Armbruster	US Air Force
	R.T. Lawn	US Army
	D.D. Rutherford	US Navy
1980–1981	R.E. Brown, M.G. Fitzpatrick, T.K. Hathaway	US Army
1981–1982	G.K. Kagawa, H.W. Robinson	US Army
	W.R. Woods	US Navy
1982–1983	J. Berger	US Air Force
	M.A. Klimt-Bianco	US Navy
	J.A. Hatten, P.A. Supon	US Army
1983–1984	J.V. Baltrukonis, J.A. Holmberg	US Navy
	K.A. Drerup	US Army
1984–1985	R.C. Platte, B.F. Sylvia	US Army
1985–1986	J.A. Schmidt, B.M. Wannamacher	US Army
	A.U. Smith	US Air Force
1986–1987	B.G. Brown-Bartley	US Navy
	W.L. Gibbs	US Air Force
	D.M. Miller, G.C. Norris	US Army

1987–1988	J.L. Bryant, D. Lofquist, L.W. Wulff-Groshell	US Air Force
	D.R. Fipps, D.J. VanRozelen	US Army
	R. Girven	US Navy
1988–1989	R. Dillon-Sylvester, D.A. Ferguson, L.E. Johansen	US Air Force
	R.A. Slater	US Navy
	N.R. Webster	US Army
1989–1990	G.D. Griffin, R. Perron, D.A. Stewart	US Army
	J. Hager, H.L. Smith	US Air Force
	C.M. Roper	US Navy
1990–1991	T. Andersen, S.E. Knoll, K.J. Markland	US Air Force
	S.E. Beardsley, E.S. Perry	US Army
	M.C. Libby	US Navy
1991–1992	C.H. Bennett, F.J. Rentas	US Army
	D.C. Davis, K.R. Holmes, F. Saraceni	US Air Force
	F.C. Music	US Navy
1992–1993	J.L. Daugirda, R. Gonzales, V.J. Welsh	US Army
	R.A. Purkhiser	US Air Force
	J.T. Scherrer	US Navy
1993–1994	M.C. Crowell	US Navy
	J.L. Giglio, R.H. McBride	US Air Force
	A.D. Hawkins, R.K. Pell Jr., H.F. Peterson	US Army
1994–1995	R.G. Alford	US Air Force
	S.E. Allen	US Navy
	E. Gourdine	US Army
1995–1996	B.G. Casleton, J.P. Ruddell	US Air Force
	S.L. Dunn, R.A. Fryar, D.T. Reiber	US Army
	A.K. Knight	US Navy
1996–1997	K.J. Belanger, H. Velazquez	US Army
	G.W. Jones, C.R. Watson	US Air Force
	F.C. Mettille	US Navy
1997–1998	R.L. Fahie, J.F. Van Patten	US Navy
	M.C. Hawkins, L.K. Viveros	US Air Force

1998–1999	B.J. Bachman, M.J. Buckellew, M.A. Sloan, R.M. Whitacre	US Army
	R.C. Davis	US Navy
	M. Montes	US Air Force
1999–2000	S.R. Futterman, A.C. Mattoch	US Air Force
2000–2001	A.M. Hudson	US Air Force
	C.C. Lelkens	Netherlands Army
	M.J. Lopatka, J.F. Quesada	US Army
	R.S. Watson	US Navy
2001–2002	S.C. Clifford	US Navy
	A.F. Colon	US Army
	G.A. Hestilow, C.L. Murphy	US Air Force
2002–2003	C.E. Bell	US Army
	K.F. Fumia, D.A. Lincoln	US Air Force
	D.H. Koch, B.K. Williamson	US Navy
2003–2004	A.J. Harding, R.D. Hayden, M.J. Roth	US Navy
	H. McDonald, A.L. Taylor	US Army
2004–2005	R.A. Borders, C.R. Jenkins	US Navy
	R.J. Curtis, R.R. Leslie-Holt, K.B. Shaw	US Air Force
	M.T. Swingholm	US Army
2005–2006	A. Cofresi, J.D. Hughes	US Air Force
	J.B. Corley, C.L. Evans, V.M. McCarthy, C.W. Mester	US Army
	J.E. Culpepper, J.A. Hoiles	US Navy
2006–2007	K.J. Buikema	US Air Force
	R.G. Gates, T.M. Terry	US Army
	F.A. Matheu, T.J. Riley	US Navy
2007–2008	A.V. Casco-Figueroa	US Army
	A.B. Polito	US Air Force
	L.E. Riggs	US Navy
	K.W. Davis	US Army Reserve*
2008–2009	J.F. Badloe	Netherlands Army
	A.R. Bartmier, S.D. Glenn	US Air Force
	D.E. Desmond	US Navy
	J. Trevino	US Army

2009-2010	W.M. Adamian, S.M. Dilworth, E.Q. Morrison	US Army
	H.A. McMinn	US Air Force
	L.A. Pecenka, J.P. Stephan	US Navy
2010-2011	M.E. Burke	US Air Force
	E. Guzman, C.I. Knaus	US Navy
	G.G. Kellar	US Army

Walter Reed National Military Medical Center, Bethesda, MD		
Year	Graduates	Service
2011-2012	J.A. Valdez, S. Golla	US Navy
	R.L. Hill	US Army
	N.M. Ferguson	US Air Force
2012-2013	M. Collins	US Navy
	C.C. Huang, S.E. McDaniel, J.M. Messenger	US Army
	E.P. Griffin, J.J. Jacobsen	US Air Force
2013-2014	T.R. Belin, M.J. Coon	US Navy
	J.L. Cheser III, J.D. Kuper, V.D. Ortiz	US Army
	B.D. Cruz	US Air Force
2014-2015	N.D. Baker, V.L. Duncan, P.B. Munerman, J.E. Guzman	US Army
	F.L. DeForrest, J.G. Hasty	US Navy
	L.A. Beeman, E.N. Robinson	US Air Force
	T.D. Puget	French Army
2015-2016	M.A. Bauldry, W.A. Ceballos	US Army
	E. Garciaperez, A.B. Brooke-Schultz	US Air Force
	J.C. Hebert	US Navy
	M. Zoodsma	Netherlands Army
2016-2017	A.M. Mott	US Army
	J.A. Bradley, L.B. King	US Air Force
	T.P. Hopkins, T.A. Reynolds	US Navy

*non-resident student (audit)
Data source: Armed Services Blood Program Office.

Throughout the distinguished history of the BBF, many senior officers have overseen it as director, including Lieutenant Colonels Joseph Akeroyd, Frank Camp, Richard Platte, Tom Hathaway, Lloyd Lippert, Patrick Supon, Mike Fitzpatrick, Mike Stanton, Stephen Beardsley, Frank Rentas, and Robert "Ken" Pell Jr. However, it wasn't just senior Army Blood Program officers who led the program. The BBF has had a civilian program director since 1976. Past directors include Jan Sigmon, LeeAnn Ziebell, Nancy Murphy, Eve Tenali, and Bill Turcan, who is director of the program as of 2016.

When Walter Reed Army Medical Center closed in September 2011 as a result of the Base Realignment and Closure Commission Act of 2005, the Blood Bank Fellowship relocated once again. Its current home is at the new Walter Reed National Military Medical Center in Bethesda, Maryland, according to Bill Turcan's email dated February 2012.

Graduates of the Fellowship

Whether in Kentucky; Washington, DC; or Maryland, the BBF has a proud history of training medical technologists from all three services to become specialists in blood banking (Figure A-3). As of early 2012, more than 175 officers from the Army, Navy, and Air Force had graduated from the program (Table A-1).

REFERENCES

1. US Department of Defense. *United States Armed Forces Medical Journal*. Washington, DC. 1959;10(9):1108.
2. US Department of the Army. *Annual Report of the Surgeon General, United States Army Fiscal Year 1965*. Washington, DC: Office of The Surgeon General; 1965.

APPENDIX B
Influential People of the Army Blood Program

Over the years, many talented individuals have made the Army Blood Program what it is today. Some have truly been pioneers in the blood banking field and have left their mark in military medical history.

Major General Douglas Kendrick, MD

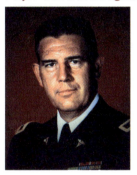

In 1940, Dr. Kendrick initiated a blood research program at the Army Medical School. He served as chief of that program until November 1944. Dr. Kendrick was also appointed to serve as the special representative on blood and plasma transfusions in the Office of The Surgeon General in 1943. Just after the war ended, he served as General Douglas MacArthur's personal physician in Japan. Dr. Kendrick became the chief surgeon of the US Army in Europe by 1960, and a few years later he authored the influential book *Blood Program in World War II*. Kendrick commanded Walter Reed Army Medical Center from 1963 until 1967, when he retired from the Army. He subsequently accepted the position of medical director at Grady Memorial Hospital in Atlanta, Georgia. Dr. Kendrick passed away in September 1994. Dr. Kendrick, whose career played a critical role in the development of the Army Blood Program, served in the Army for more than 33 years. The blood donor center at the Dwight D. Eisenhower Army Medical Center at Ft Gordon, Georgia, was dedicated in his honor in May 2001. (Photo courtesy of the Kendrick Memorial Blood Center, Ft Gordon, Georgia.)

Colonel Joseph H. Akeroyd, MD

Colonel Akeroyd began his Army service in 1943 as a clinical laboratory officer and biochemist. He served in the European Theater of Operations with the

178th, 197th, and 124th General Hospitals during World War II. In 1947 he was assigned to Brooke General Hospital, where he most notably researched and tested plastic blood collection bags. From 1957 to 1958, Colonel Akeroyd served as the Army representative to the task force on military blood collecting. To ensure well-trained officers in all phases of blood banking, he established the US Army blood bank fellowship program at Walter Reed Army Institute of Research in Washington, DC, in 1958. While assigned to the institute, Colonel Akeroyd served as the chief of immunology. He determined the blood type of Abraham Lincoln (type A), from blood samples preserved at the Armed Forces Institute of Pathology. The samples came from the cuffs of 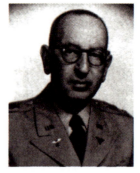 one of the physicians tending to Lincoln after he was shot. Colonel Akeroyd returned to Brooke General Hospital in 1961 and served as chief of the blood bank until his death in September 1963. The blood donor center at Ft Sam Houston was renamed the Akeroyd Blood Donor Center in 1993 to honor one of the most influential people in the Army Blood Program. (Photo reproduced from Camp FR, Conte N, Brewer JR. *Military Blood Banking 1941-1973– Lessons Learned Applicable to Civil Disasters and Other Considerations.* Ft Knox, Kentucky: US Army Medical Research Laboratory; 1973: ix.)

Lieutenant Colonel William S. Collins II

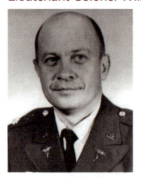

Lieutenant Colonel Collins (BBF class of '58–59) is one of the most influential men in the Army Blood Program's history. As a first lieutenant, he was selected to be the first official student in the US Army BBF. His career shaped the way blood could be shipped to service members overseas. The Vietnam War will be remembered for many things, among them the introduction of the Styrofoam blood box, which was introduced by Major Collins in 1965. The Collins box enabled the shipping of blood at required temperatures, regardless of the temperature outside. It was easier to handle, was less susceptible to damage, and was far less expensive than the cardboard inserts used earlier. According to Neel, Collins "received $935 for his suggestion, and his innovation resulted in a first-year savings of $56,000 and a new flexibility in military blood banking."[1] (Photo courtesy of Mr. Bill Turcan, US Army Blood Bank Fellowship.)

Colonel Frank R. Camp

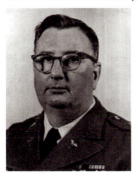

Colonel Camp (BBF class of '60–61) is known as the father of the Armed Services Blood Program (ASBP). Over the course of his influential 32-year career, Colonel Camp was a major force in shaping the Army Blood Program. On July 1, 1965, Colonel Camp became the first director of the blood transfusion research division at the US Army Medical Research Laboratory at Ft Knox, where he is known for improving the way blood was shipped and transfused. He served there until 1975. Recognized and highly respected worldwide for his blood banking and transfusion research, Colonel Camp was a contributor to the 5th and 6th editions of the AABB's *Technical Methods and Procedures* manual covering 1970 through 1974. During that same 4-year period, Colonel Camp served on the AABB's standards committee. He was also an adjunct associate professor of biology at Bowling Green State University, Ohio. The AABB awarded Colonel Camp the distinguished service award in 1973. Upon his retirement from the Army in 1974, Colonel Camp continued his work in the field as scientific director/director of the Louisville Regional Red Cross Blood Center. He retired from the American Red Cross in 1980. Colonel Camp passed away on April 14, 1983. One year later, in July 1984, the blood bank center at Ft Knox was renamed the Colonel Frank R. Camp Memorial Blood Center in honor of this great Army Blood Program pioneer. Colonel Camp was posthumously awarded the ASBP Lifetime Achievement Award in 2012. (Photograph from Camp Memorial Blood Center, Ft Knox, Kentucky, closure files, courtesy of the Army Blood Program Office.)

Lieutenant Colonel A. Matthew Gottlieb

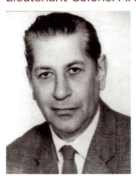

Lieutenant Colonel Gottlieb (BBF class of '61–62) was a contributor to the 4th edition of the AABB's *Technical Methods and Procedures* manual in 1966. He was active in the South Central Association of Blood Banks, serving as the organization's president in 1971. Years later the association named one of their awards in honor of Lieutenant Colonel Gottlieb—the Dr. Matthew Gottlieb Rising Star Award. In 1992, Lieutenant Colonel Gottlieb published *A Pictorial History of Blood Practices and Transfusions*. (Photo courtesy of Mr. Bill Turcan, US Army Blood Bank Fellowship.)

Colonel James Spiker Jr.

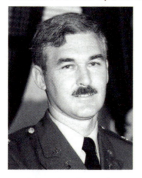

The illustrious military blood banking career of Colonel Spiker (BBF class of '65–66) is filled with firsts. He served as the first Health Services Command (HSC) clinical laboratory and blood bank consultant, and he developed requirements for all HSC blood banks to be both accredited by the AABB and licensed by the Food and Drug Administration (FDA). He further coordinated and performed pre-inspection consultant visits to all HSC sites to prepare for FDA licensing of blood products, thereby making a major contribution to the safety and integrity of the military blood supply. Colonel Spiker also promoted and directed the conversion of triservice military blood bank manuals into official AABB manuals. In 1979 he transferred to the Office of The Surgeon General in Falls Church, Virginia, where he established and served as the first director of the US Army Blood Program—the first official Army-wide blood program. He also served as the laboratory sciences consultant to the surgeon general. Colonel Spiker set up the first Army additional skill identifier (8T) to ensure authorized positions for blood bank officers and served as the Army Blood Program officer from 1979 to 1990. Colonel Spiker also served as chief of medical allied sciences and assistant chief for the Medical Service Corps from May 1983 to August 1990, according to Colonel (Retired) Anthony Polk's email dated August 2010. Spiker received the ASBP Lifetime Achievement Award at the annual AABB meeting in San Diego, California, in 2011. (Photo courtesy of Colonel [Ret] James Spiker Jr.)

Colonel Anthony Polk

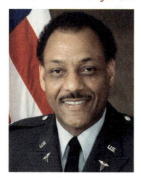

Colonel Polk (BBF class of '72–73) was another important leader in the Army Blood Program. Throughout his 25-year career, Colonel Polk served at various levels within the Army Blood Program. However, he is primarily recognized for his work in the joint environment of the ASBP, where he served as the director from 1984 to 1991. He authored The Military Blood Program 2004 Implementation Plan to establish blood program goals and resources. The plan's inclusion in the DoD's Medical Readiness Strategic Plan, approved by the secretary of defense, marked the beginning of the military blood program's routine inclusion in all contingency plans. Subsequent participation in all worldwide military exercises trained personnel at all levels on

ASBP operations in wartime. He also coordinated and implemented the world's largest frozen blood program, adding frozen blood product depots around the world on land and ships.

To reflect the importance and triservice nature of the military blood program, Colonel Polk changed the name of the Military Blood Program Office to the Armed Services Blood Program Office and coined the titles "service blood program officer," "joint blood program officer," and "area joint blood program officer." He developed a one-page worldwide distribution system for all unified commands that included standardized terms and a distribution system scheme. Colonel Polk also oversaw the first wartime frozen blood operation, during Operation Desert Storm; added a noncommissioned officer and two field grade officers to the Armed Services Blood Program Office staff; and developed a monthly class for new blood bank fellows—still in use today—to give new blood bankers on-the-ground skills. Colonel Polk served on the AABB's Standards Committee from 1987 through 1991. Colonel Polk received the ASBP Lifetime Achievement Award at the AABB Annual meeting in New Orleans, Louisiana, in October 2009. (Photo courtesy of Colonel [Ret] Anthony Polk.)

Colonel Richard Brown

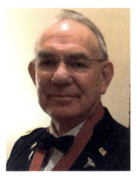

Colonel Brown (BBF class of '80–81) was a visionary who saw a future blood program in which triservice staffing and triservice blood resource sharing became the norm, a future in which computers replaced paper records, and FDA licensure and quality assurance became overriding principles for survival in a competitive blood bank industry. As the laboratory manager at Ft Ord Medical Activity, he built a viable blood collection program that laid the groundwork for the first multiservice blood bank, the Armed Services Blood Bank Center. As the commander of the 655th Medical Company (US Army Europe Blood Bank) in Germany in June 1987, Colonel Brown oversaw the implementation of the HIV testing program for all Army blood collecting facilities in Europe. He also coordinated the roll out of HIV testing and the availability of tested blood products with his colleagues at US Air Force Europe and Navy Europe, according to Colonel (Retired) Frank Rentas' email dated September 2014. Colonel Brown served as director of the Army Blood Program from 1991 through 1997. He guided the Army Blood Program through a dynamic period of change in the US blood industry, when the FDA exerted its authority over the industry and enforced the regulation of blood as a pharmaceutical (instead of a biologic). When the FDA implemented its current good manufacturing practices and quality plan regulations, Colonel Brown shepherded this major cultural change. He created the quality assurance manager position for the Army Blood Program in September 1995. He and the quality assurance manager began conducting regular facility audits, publishing audit reports for senior leadership's awareness, and making inroads into standardizing operating procedures. He reorganized the Army's FDA license structure and ensured all blood collection sites obtained FDA licensure. Colonel Brown was accountable for the Army Blood Program as the first alternate responsible head, a position required for FDA blood establishment licensing. As director, he rewrote and published the Army Blood Program regulations. Many admired Colonel Brown because he took time to really get to know and mentor the officers, soldiers, and civilians who worked in the program, according to Kathleen Elder's email dated July 2011. (Photo courtesy of Colonel [Ret] Richard Brown.)

Colonel Richard Platte

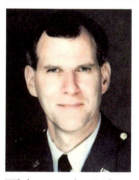

In 1978, as a young laboratory officer, Colonel Platte (BBF class of '84–85) revitalized the Korea Area Blood Program after it had been absorbed into the 121st Evacuation Hospital. After several years of rebuilding its teams and reconstituting its equipment, the program participated in Team Spirit 1982. The increase in HIV and AIDS in the mid-1980s ushered in the most remarkable change that the Army Blood Program had encountered since the introduction of plastic collection bags. While assigned to Walter Reed Army Medical Center, Colonel Platte performed the very first HTLV-III test in April 1985. With new infectious disease testing requirements and look-back investigations, blood banking became increasingly complicated. Colonel Platte became a driving force in the effort to bring computerization to the Army Blood Program. He participated on a task force created to begin building the Defense Blood Management Information System in April 1987. As the HSC laboratory and blood bank consultant, he found the HIV look-back effort inadequate and convinced the HSC commander to increase efforts and resources to build a more robust program to centrally manage the ever increasing number of cases. His final assignment was serving as the executive officer of the Armed Forces Institute of Pathology. (Photo courtesy of Colonel [Ret] Richard Platte.)

Kathleen Elder

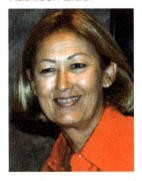

Ms. Elder was the first quality assurance manager for the Army Blood Program, serving from September 1995 through November 2012. During a time of tremendous change in the blood industry, Ms. Elder quickly began building a quality assurance and self-assessment plan for the Army Blood Program to ensure that every transfusion service and blood donor center in the Army Medical Command (MEDCOM) were consistent with the required principles of quality assurance and current good manufacturing practices. She initiated a series of workshops that inspired all MEDCOM transfusion services and blood donor centers to achieve a higher level of quality in manufacturing blood products and performing transfusion services. Shortly thereafter, Ms. Elder began a program of facility audits to help sites exceed the FDA's federal regulatory requirements and AABB accreditation standards. Her efforts ensured that every MEDCOM facility consistently received high results on outside agency inspections. In 2006 Ms. Elder led a standardization initiative of processes and procedures across the Army Blood Program, which fit well with the Army Blood Program Office's long-standing commitment to improving quality, operational efficiency, and regulatory compliance across the program. She represented the DoD as a member of the AABB Accreditation Committee for many years. She enjoyed mentoring individuals on all aspects of quality management and frequently provided presentations at various venues. (Photo courtesy of the Army Blood Program Office.)

Colonel Noel Webster

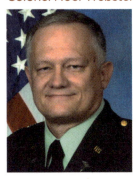

Colonel Webster (BBF class of '88–89) was selected to attend the resident course for the Command and General Staff College in 1991—the only ASBPO officer ever chosen to attend in residence. He subsequently served 5 years at the ASBP office, 3 years as deputy director of modernization, and 2 years as deputy director for operations. He coauthored chapter 15, "Military Transfusion Practice," in the Textbook of Military Medicine *Anesthesia and Perioperative Care of the Combat Casualty* in 1995. Colonel Webster was a contributor to the 12th edition of the AABB's Technical Manual in 1996. Colonel Webster served as director of clinical laboratory programs and consultant for laboratory services for the surgeon general from 2001 through 2006. The Medical Service Corps chief chose Colonel Webster as the assistant corps chief of allied health sciences for 2007 through 2008. After 9/11, Colonel Webster was instrumental in implementing a new biosecurity program that included regional biosafety level 3 testing capabilities. He was a member of the MEDCOM technology and assessment and requirements analysis team. Through his dedication and hard work, the team was awarded the Surgeon General Excalibur award in 2003.

Colonel Webster implemented the Six Sigma program in the MEDCOM laboratory program, resulting in more than 20 black belt, 40 green belt, and 140 yellow belt recipients, and over 20 projects and more than $6 million in savings and improved quality. He and his team received the Surgeon General Excalibur award in 2007 for this program. From August 2004 to February 2005, as part of the newly formed Multinational Forces–Iraq headquarters surgeon's office, Colonel Webster was the Iraq Area Joint Blood Program officer. He also was a liaison with the US Department of State and with the Iraq ministry of health. He worked closely with the ministry of health's director of operations and his director of blood banking by assisting them in designing new blood bank centers. He was the acting medical liaison to the ministry of health during the Fallujah Battle of 2004. He worked closely with the minister of health and the deputy commander of Multi-National Forces–Iraq to ensure the displaced population of Fallujah was getting necessary medical, food, and survival care. He was also instrumental in setting up written approved guidance from the chief of staff of the Iraqi government on the burial policy for Iraqi people and enemy combatants killed in the Fallujah battle. Colonel Webster was selected in August 2006 to become the deputy chief of staff at MEDCOM. (Photo courtesy of the Robertson Blood Center, Ft Hood, Texas.)

Colonel Elaine Perry

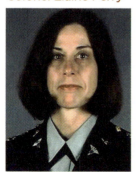

Colonel Perry (BBF class of '90–91) served as chief of the blood bank and hematology branch of the Academy of Health Sciences at the Army Medical Center and School from August 1977 through July 2000. She instituted the DoD user and system administrator courses for the Defense Blood Standard System. Colonel Perry directed the largest and most productive blood center in the DoD, Robertson Blood Center at Ft Hood, from July 2000 through July 2004. While director, she also served as the primary investigator for all 25 DoD donor centers' nucleic acid testing protocols for HIV/HCV and West Nile virus. She participated in the joint Public Health

Service and FDA nucleic acid testing working group for blood donation policy and practice. In 2004 she became the first female clinical laboratory blood program officer to be selected for promotion to the rank of colonel. (Photo courtesy of the Robertson Blood Center, Ft Hood, Texas.)

Colonel Donna Whittaker

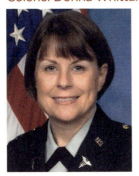

In 2002 Colonel Whittaker designed the modern bloodmobile, which is now in use at Brooke Army Medical Center and served as the prototype for a bloodmobile that was purchased for all Army blood donor centers. As a blood program officer, she started the Six Sigma program for all clinical laboratory and blood program officers in 2004. The Army surgeon general awarded her the Excalibur award for launching the War on Waste Six Sigma business initiative, which saved more than $1.6 million in the first year. Later, she became the Army Medical Department's first certified Lean Six Sigma master black belt. She was honored with the DoD's science, technology, engineering, and math award in 2002. In 2009 Colonel Whittaker became the first female and first blood program officer to hold the position of dean of the Academy of Health Sciences at the Army Medical Department Center and School. (Photo courtesy of Army Medical Department Center and School, Ft Sam Houston, Texas.)

Colonel Audra Taylor

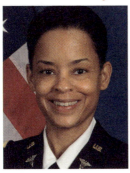

Colonel Taylor (BBF class of '03–04) became the first female director of the Army Blood Program in 2014. Her years and breadth of experience made her the ideal person to serve as the 10th director. She activated the 432nd Blood Support Detachment at Ft Bragg and served as the unit's first commander until July 2008. In 2009, she deployed with Task Force 28th Combat Support Hospital, where she served as the Chief, Blood Services and as the theater laboratory consultant in support of Operation Iraqi Freedom. After redeploying back to Ft Sam Houston, she served as the first program director for the consolidated (Army and Navy) Medical Laboratory Technician Course at the Medical Education and Training Campus. Colonel Taylor deployed in September 2013 as the US Central Command Joint Blood Program Officer Forward, in support of Operation Enduring Freedom.

After many years of preparatory work by colleagues, Colonel Taylor's support culminated in several of the Army blood donor centers receiving bloodmobiles. Traditionally, blood donor centers had a van of mobile donor beds and supply chests, and would set up operations with sponsoring military units provided they had sufficient space and proper climate control. These requirements made it almost impossible to collect donors in locations such as motor pools, in-processing centers, post exchanges, or commissaries. The advantage of the bloodmobile is that they can go into high density population areas and collect blood. The required space and proper climate is all contained within the bloodmobile. (Photo courtesy of Colonel [Ret] Audra Taylor.)

REFERENCES
1. Neel SH. *Medical Support of the US Army in Vietnam 1965–1970*. Washington, DC: Department of the Army; 1991.

APPENDIX C
Complete List of Army Blood Program Leaders

Table C-1. Directors of the Army Blood Program

Tenure	Name
1979–1990	COL James Spiker Jr.
1991–1997	COL Richard Brown
1997–2000	COL Gary Kagawa
2000–2001	LTC Dennis Stewart
2001–2005	COL Gary Norris
2005–2008	COL Steven Beardsley
2008–2009	LTC Michael Lopatka
2009–2012	COL Ronny Fryar
2012–2014	COL Richard Gonzales
2104–present	COL Audra Taylor

COL: Colonel; LTC: Lieutenant Colonel

Data source: Army Blood Program Office.

Table C-2. Health Services Command laboratory and blood bank consultants

Tenure	Name
1974–1979	LTC James Spiker Jr.
1979–1985	COL Robert "Bob" Usry
1985–1988	LTC Gerald "Jerry" Jacobs
1988–1993	COL Richard Platte

COL: Colonel; LTC: Lieutenant Colonel

Data source: Army Blood Program Office.

Table C-3. Army Officers assigned to the Military Blood Program Agency Armed Services Blood Program Office

Tenure	Name
1962–1964	LTC Edward O'Shaughnessy, MC*
1964–1966	LTC William Leslie, MC*
1966–1971	COL Richard Krakaur, MC*
1971–1972	COL James McCarthy, MC*
1972–1973	COL Janice Mendelson, MC*
1973–1975	LTC Turman Allen, MS
1975–1977	COL Bob Angel[†‡]
1977–1978	COL Doug Beach[†§]
1979–1981	LTC Jim Spiker[†¥]
1982–1984	COL Jim Spiker[†¥]
1984–1991	COL Anthony Polk, MS*
1992–1997	LTC Noel Webster, MS
1997–1999	LTC G. Michael Fitzpatrick, MS
1999–2003	COL G. Michael Fitzpatrick, MS*
2003–2006	LTC Ronny Fryar, MS
2006–2008	LTC Michael Lopatka, MS
2008–2012	COL Frank Rentas, MS*
2012–2015	LTC Jason Corley, MS
2015–present	LTC Carmen Bell, MS

LTC: Lieutenant Colonel; COL: Colonel; MC: Medical Corps; MS: Medical Service Corps

* Denotes director
† Because blood requirements outside the continental United States were low in the post-Vietnam era, Military Blood Program Office staffing authorizations were reduced to one officer (director), one noncommissioned officer, and one secretary. (According to Colonel [Retired] James Spiker, when either an Air Force or Navy officer was the director, an Army officer was assigned additional duty as the Army deputy director.)
‡ Colonel Angel was a biochemist and laboratory consultant at the Office of The Surgeon General. He was also chief for medical allied sciences and assistant chief of the Medical Services Corps.
§ Colonel Beach was a biochemist at Ft Detrick and also acting laboratory consultant at the Office of The Surgeon General. He was detailed to work a couple of days each week at the Military Blood Program Office.
¥ Lieutenant Colonel James Spiker was the point of contact for "blood bank specific" information for Colonel Beach and Colonel Angel (COL [Ret] Jim Spiker, Personal Communication, 24 March, 2104).

Data Source: Army Blood Program Office.

Table C-4. Army Medical Department Blood Program consultants*

Tenure	Name
1991–1998	COL Richard Brown
1998–2001	COL G. Michael Fitzpatrick
2001–2005	COL Gary Norris
2005–2008	COL Steven Beardsley
2009–2012	COL Ronny Fryar
2012–2014	COL Richard Gonzales

COL: Colonel

* In Fall 2014, Army Medical Department senior leaders conducted a review of all surgeon general consultant positions with the goal of reducing the number. Specialty consultants were rolled under related Area of Concentration consultants. The respective corps chiefs approved the recommended reductions. Colonel Richard Gonzales was the last blood program consultant. On his retirement, the blood program consultant responsibilities rolled under the clinical laboratory science consultant.

Data Source: Army Blood Program Office.

Table C-5. Army Blood Program officers supporting other military operations

Military Operation	Name
Operation Just Cause (Panama) 1989–1990	MAJ Mike Stanton (AJBPO) 32nd Medical Command
Operation Restore Hope (Somalia) 1992–1993	MAJ Jeff Schmidt (AJBPO) Blood Platoon, 32nd Medical Logistics Battalion
Operation Uphold Democracy (Haiti) 1994–1995	MAJ Joanne Daugirda Blood Platoon, 32nd Medical Logistics Battalion
Operations Joint Endeavor, Joint Guard, Joint Forge (Bosnia)* 1996–2004 USEUCOM JBPOs	MAJ Robert "Ken" Pell MAJ Ronny Fryar MAJ Dave Reiber MAJ Robin Whitacre MAJ Robert "Ken" Pell
Operation Joint Guardian (Kosovo)† 1999–current USEUCOM JBPOs	MAJ Ronny Fryar MAJ Dave Reiber MAJ Robin Whitacre MAJ Robert "Ken" Pell MAJ Jose Quesada LTC Robin Whittaker MAJ Matthew Swingholm
Operation Unified Endeavor (Haiti earthquake response) 2010	MAJ Christopher Evans 153rd Blood Support Detachment

MAJ: Major; AJBPO: Area Joint Blood Program Officer; USEUCOM: US European Command

* The blood platoon from the 226th Medical Logistics Battalion deployed early in the Bosnia operation. Lieutenant Wendy Sammons and Lieutenant Jon Davis were two of the platoon leaders. As the operation stabilized and downsized, the blood platoon redeployed and the staff of the combat support hospital laboratory functioned as the blood supply unit.

† Because of the medical footprint in Kosovo, US European Command did not deploy a blood support unit or blood transshipment center in the area of operation. Blood products were provided by military donor centers across Europe. The blood was shipped to the US Army Europe Blood Donor Center, which also received supplements from the continental United States. The blood was then shipped directly to the 212th Mobile Army Surgical Hospital.

Data Source: Army Blood Program Office.

APPENDIX D
US Army Blood Donor Infectious Disease Testing

Table D-1. Timeline of infectious disease testing of blood donors in the US Army

Date	Test
Early 1940s	Kahn test for syphilis*
1946	VDRL test for syphilis
1961	RPR test for syphilis
1971	HBsAg
1985	Anti-HIV
1986	Anti-HBc
1987	ALT
1989	Anti-HTLV-1
1990	Anti-HCV (v. 1.0)
1992	Anti-HIV-1/HIV-2
1992	Anti-HCV (v. 2.0)
1995	ALT testing ends
1995	HIV-p24 antigen
1997	Anti-HTLV-1/2
2000	Single Donor HIV and HCV NAT under IND
2002	FDA licenses single-donor HIV and HCV NAT
2002	HIV-p24 antigen testing ends
2003	WNV NAT under IND
2007	FDA licenses WNV NAT
2011	Anti-T. cruzi (Chagas disease)
2016	Zika virus NAT under IND

VDRL: venereal disease research laboratory; RPR: rapid plasma reagin; HBsAG: hepatitis B surface antigen test; anti: antigen; HIV: human immunodeficiency virus; HBc: hepatitis B core antigen; ALT: alanine aminotransferase; HTLV; humant T-lymphotropic virus; HCV: hepatitis C virus; NAT: nucleic acid test; IND: investigational new drug; FDA: Food and Drug Administration; WNV: West Nile virus

*Serologic tests for syphilis were developed in the early 1900s. The Kahn test was developed in 1922. With 138 cases of transfusion transmitted syphilis being documented by 1941, testing donor blood for syphilis began.

Data source: Army Blood Program Office.

Acronyms and Abbreviations

A
AABB: American Association of Blood Banks
ABC: American Blood Commission
ABCC: ASBPO Blood Coordinating Committee
ABP: Army Blood Program
ABPO: Army Blood Program office/officer
ACD: acid-citrate-dextrose AABB
AFB: Air Force Base
AIDS: acquired immunodeficiency syndrome
ALT: alanine aminotransferase liver test
AMEDD: Army Medical Department
AMEDDC&S: Army Medical Department Center and School
AR: Army regulation
ARC: American Red Cross
AS-1: Adsol (Fenwal Inc, Lake Zurich, IL)
AS-3: Nutricel (Cutter Biological, Berkeley, CA)
AS-5: Optisol (Terumo Corp, Tokyo, Japan)
ASBBC: Armed Services Blood Bank Center
ASBP: Armed Services Blood Program
ASBPO: Armed Services Blood Program Office
ASD(HA): assistant secretary of defense for health affairs
ASWBPL: Armed Services Whole Blood Processing Laboratory
ATP: adenosine triphosphate

B
BAMC: Brooke Army Medical Center
BBF: Blood Bank Fellowship
BDC: blood donor center
BRAC: base realignment and closure
BSD: blood support detachment
BSE: bovine spongiform encephalopathy

C
CASEVAC: casualty evacuation
CBRNE: chemical, biological, radiological, nuclear, explosive
CCMRF: CBRNE consequence management response force
CENTCOM: Central Command
CFR: case fatality rate; Code of Federal Regulations
CJD: Creutzfeldt-Jakob disease
CONUS: continental United States
CPD: citrate-phosphate-dextrose
CPDA-1: citrate phosphate dextrose adenine
CP2D: citrate-phosphate-double-dextrose

D
DBMIS: Defense Blood Management Information System
DBSS: Defense Blood Standard System
DCRF: defense chemical, biological, radiological, and nuclear (CBRN) response force
DD: Department of Defense (eg, DD Form)
DEPMEDS: deployable medical systems
DNA: deoxyribonucleic acid
DoD: Department of Defense

E
ELISA: enzyme-linked immunosorbent assay
EMEDS: expeditionary medical support
ETOUSA: European Theater of Operations, United States Army
EUCOM: European Command

F
FDA: Food and Drug Administration
FWB: fresh whole blood

H
HBV: hepatitis B virus
HCV: hepatitis C virus
HIV: human immunodeficiency virus
HSC: Health Services Command
HTLV: human T-cell lymphotropic virus

I
IND: investigational new drug

J
JBPO: joint blood program officer

M
MBP: Military Blood Program
MBPA: Military Blood Program Agency
MBPO: Military Blood Program Office
MDBS: medical detachment, blood support
MEDCOM: Medical Command
MEDEVAC: medical evacuation
MOS: military occupational specialty
MOU: memorandum of understanding
MRSP: medical readiness strategic plan
MSC: Medical Service Corps
MSU: medical support unit
MTF: military treatment facility
MTOE: Modified Table of Organization and Equipment
MUST: medical unit self-contained transportable

N
NAT: nucleic acid testing
NBC: National Broadcasting Company
NCOIC: noncommissioned officer in charge

O
OIF: Operation Iraqi Freedom
OTSG: Office of The Surgeon General

P
PACOM: Pacific Command
PIPA: pyruvate, inosine, phosphate, and adenine

R
RNA: ribonucleic acid
RPR: rapid plasma reagin
RT2D2: rapid transfusion transmitted disease diagnostic

S
SD: solvent and detergent
SOS: advance blood depot

T
TDA: Table of Distribution and Allowances
TMDS: Theater Medical Data Store
TRADOC: Training and Doctrine Command

U
UD: universal donor
UN: United Nations
USAMEDCOMEUR: US Army Medical Command Europe
USAREUR: US Army Europe

V
vCJD: variant Creutzfeldt-Jakob disease
VDRL: venereal disease research laboratory

W
WB PRD: whole blood pathogen reduction device
WRAMC: Walter Reed Army Medical Center

Index

A

AABB, 51, 52, 57, 59–60, 106, 132, 170, 201–202
Abbott Laboratories, 55, 56, 108, 187
ABCC. *See* Armed Services Blood Program Blood Coordinating Committee
Aberdeen Proving Ground, Maryland, 77
ABP. *See* Army Blood Program
ABPO. *See* Army Blood Program Office
Accreditation, 57, 59–62
ACD. *See* Acid-citrate-dextrose anticoagulant
Acid-citrate-dextrose anticoagulant, 5, 62
ACP215, 145, 146, 168, 170
Acquired immune deficiency syndrome, 85–87, 106, 216
Adamian, Wendy, 176
Additive solutions, 82, 176
Adsol, 82, 84
Adviento, Jocelyn, 192
Agiliu, Louis, 34
AIDS. *See* Acquired immune deficiency syndrome
Air Force Blood Transshipment Center, 159
Akeroyd, Joseph H., 5, 6, 201, 211–212
Alanine aminotransferase liver test, 84, 107
Albert, Specialist 4th Class, 40
Allen, Turman, 60
Alley, Jack, 192
Alsever's solution, 2, 5
ALT. *See* Alanine aminotransferase liver test
AMEDD. *See* Army Medical Department
AMEDDC&S. *See* Army Medical Department Center and School
American Association of Blood Banks, 52, 57, 59–60, 106, 132, 170, 201–202

American Blood Commission, 52
American Blood Commission Codabar, 123
American National Red Cross, 29
American Red Cross
    Compass program, 75
    Korean War efforts, 9
    World War II efforts, 2, 5
Aminotransferase liver test, 84
Angel, Colonel Charles, 60
Anticoagulants
    acid-citrate-dextrose, 5, 62
    citrate phosphate dextrose, 57, 62, 82
ARC. *See* American Red Cross
Armed Forces Blood Donor Program, 6–9, 10, 14–22
Armed Forces Institute of Pathology, 100
Armed Services Blood Bank Center, 77, 99
Armed Services Blood Bank Center-Pacific Northwest, 120, 122
Armed Services Blood Program, 74, 80–81
Armed Services Blood Program Blood Coordinating Committee, 78, 79
Armed Services Blood Program Office, 80, 86, 94, 102, 104, 125–126, 134, 222
Armed Services Joint Medical Planning School, 79
Armed Services Medical Material Coordinating Committee, 28
Armed Services Medical Regulating Service Office, 79–80
Armed Services Medical Regulating System, 79–80
Armed Services Whole Blood Processing Laboratory, 32, 34–38, 52, 61, 97, 149, 151
Army Blood Bank Fellowship, 27, 34, 201–210

Army Blood Program
    accreditation and licensure efforts, 59–62, 82–84
    Base Realignment and Closure Commission mandates, 99–101
    blood donations in the Military District, Washington DC, 75, 77
    blood support detachments, 189, 191–192
    blood support units, 181–193
    Compass program, 75
    directors, 221
    during early 1960s, 25–30
    facilities modernization, 174
    facility status in the early 1990s, 93–94
    foundations of the modern program, 57–58
    future improvements, 177–178
    impact of global emerging infectious diseases, 173–174
    information assurance, 172–173
    information technology, 110–111, 159–161, 172–173
    Korean War efforts, 5–12
    manufacturing requirements, 124–130
    officers supporting other military operations, 224
    operational coordination, 25–41
    Operations Desert Shield/Desert Storm efforts, 94–99
    Operations Enduring Freedom/Iraqi Freedom/New Dawn efforts, 133–158
    organizational command and control of, 57, 58
    oversight of, 62
    performance initiatives, 122–124
    post-Cold War review, 102–105
    post-Vietnam War efforts, 51–57
    process standardization, 25–41
    program growth, 25–41
    program leaders, 221–224
    program leadership in the early 1990s, 93–94
    quality assurance initiatives, 105–111, 122–124
    research and development role, 174–176
    restructuring during early 2000's, 117–121
    screening requirements, 124–130
    strategy adjustment, 157–172
    testing advances, 105–110, 124–130
    timeline, xiii–xiv
    Vietnam War efforts, 30–41
    World War II efforts, 1–5
Army Blood Program Office, 100, 106
Army Clinical Laboratory Program, 122
Army Knowledge Online, 167
Army Medical Department, 57, 97, 100, 102, 223
Army Medical Department Center and School, 34–35
Army Medical Graduate School, 6
Army Medical Research Laboratory, 29
Army Medical Service Mobilization Plan, 29
Army Support Command units, 27
AS-1, 82
AS-3, 82
AS-5, 82
AS-7, 176
ASBBC. *See* Armed Services Blood Bank Center
ASBP. *See* Armed Services Blood Program
ASBPO. *See* Armed Services Blood Program Office
ASWBPL. *See* Armed Services Whole Blood Processing Laboratory
Australian Red Cross, 5

B

Bachman, Barbara, 122, 123, 147, 148, 157
Baker, Jerry, 78
Baker, Gerald, 80
Baker, Nathan, 192
BAMC. *See* Brooke Army Medical Center
Barcoding system, 123
Barker, Dr. Lou, 60
Base Realignment and Closure Act, 99
Base Realignment and Closure Commission, 93, 99–101
Bates, James, 78
Bauldy, Manuela, 191
Bautista, Lieutenant, 158
Baxter, Sheila, 120, 122
Baxter Laboratories, 1, 5
BBF. *See* Blood Bank Fellowship
Beardsley, Stephen, 117, 118, 120, 123, 124
Belanger, Kevin, 159, 161, 176, 191
Bell, John, 37, 85, 95

Berry, Honorable Frank B., 28
Blood Bank, 30–31, 32, 36–37, 39–41
Blood Bank Bleeding Detachments, 182
Blood Bank Center, 50, 55, 81–82, 206
Blood Bank Fellowship, 27, 34, 201–210
"Blood Boxers," 149
Blood collection, storage and distribution
    early 1960s, 25–30
    Korean War efforts, 5–12
    modernization during early 2000's, 117–121
    Operations Desert Shield/Desert Storm efforts, 94–99
    Operations Enduring Freedom/Iraqi Freedom/New Dawn efforts, 133–158
    post-Cold War review, 102–105
    post-Vietnam War efforts, 51–62
    during the 1980s, 75–77
    strategy adjustment, 157–172
    Vietnam War efforts, 30–41
    World War II efforts, 1–5
Blood Coordinating Committee, 78, 79, 104
Blood donation record, 25–26, 111, 170, 171
Blood Donor Campaign, 9, 16–19
Blood Donor Procurement Program, 29
Blood Donor Program, Armed Forces, 6–9, 10, 14–22
Blood Donor Record Card, 25–26, 111
Blood donor testing, 84–87, 95, 107, 109, 168, 169, 173–174, 225–226
Blood Information Program, 159, 161
Blood preservation
    acid-citrate-dextrose anticoagulant, 5
    Alsever's solution, 2
Blood Program. *See* Army Blood Program
Blood Program in World War II, 29
Blood shipping box, 31, 32, 33
Blood shipping container, 141, 143–144
Blood support detachments, 189, 191–192
Blood support units, 181–193
Blood Transfusion Division, 34, 202
Blood transfusion service, 29
Blood Transfusion Units, 181
Blood typing, 104, 145, 147
Bolan, Charles, 141
Borowski, Robert, 94, 185
Boutte, Judy, 133
Bovine spongiform encephalopathy, 124–125

Bowling Green State University, Ohio, 202–204
BRAC. *See* Base Realignment and Closure Commission
Brewer, Jerry, 34, 55, 57, 185
Brooke Army Medical Center, 52, 55, 61–62, 109
Brooke Army Medical Center Blood Donor Center, 34–35
Brown, Richard, 93, 100, 107, 109–111, 124, 185, 186, 204, 215–216
BSDs. *See* Blood support detachments
BSE. *See* Bovine spongiform encephalopathy
Buckellew, Mike, 156
Bukovitz, Mike, 157
Bush, George H.W., 94
Bush, George W., 131, 134, 136

C

Camp, Frank R., 29, 34, 55, 57, 180, 200, 202, 213
Camp Memorial Blood Center, 81, 96, 110, 118
Campos, Crista, 158
Cap, Andre, 177 Cardiolipin microflocculation tests, 27 Carodine, Joretha, 133
Cascofigeroa, Aleskey, 191
CASEVAC. *See* casualty evacuation
Casualty Evacuation, 151
Ceballos, William, 158, 191
Central Command, 94, 97, 133–137, 151, 154–155, 159
Chagas disease, 173
Cheser, Joseph, III, 158, 192
Chiron Corporation, 129
Cho, John, 171
Citrate phosphate dextrose adenine, 57, 62, 82
Citrate phosphate-double dextrose, 82
Civil defense, 9
CJD. *See* Creutzfeldt-Jakob disease
Clayton, Roderick, 157
Clinical Laboratory Improvement Amendments of 1988, 102–103
Clinton, Dr. Jarrett, 126, 128
Codabar, 123
Cold War
    post-war review of Army Blood Program, 102–105
Coley, Herbert, 171

Collins, William S., II, 30, 31, 184–185, 202, 212
Collins box, 31, 32, 33, 97
Colon, Major Angel, 120, 122
Combat Application Tourniquet, 144
Commission on Accreditation of Allied Health Education Programs, 201
Compass program, 75
Composite Resources Inc., 144
Container Delivery Drop, 188
Conte, Colonel Nicholas, 55, 57
Cooley, Private First Class, 40
Corley, Jason, 156, 158, 177, 191
Cosgrove, Todd, 173
CPDA-1. *See* Citrate phosphate dextrose adenine
Craig Joint Theater Hospital, 147
Creutzfeldt-Jakob disease, 124–128
Crosby, William H., 6, 28, 29, 201–202
Crouch, Madge, 60
Cryoprecipitate, 62, 139, 141,
Cuban missile crisis, 28

D

Davis, Kenneth, 118, 120, 137, 172
DBMIS. *See* Defense Blood Management Information System
DBSS. *See* Defense Blood Standard System
DD Form 572, 25–26, 170, 171
Defense Blood Management Information System, 86, 110
Defense Blood Standard System, 86, 110, 167, 172
Defense Health Headquarters, 171
Defense Medical Logistics Standard Support, 110
Defense Medical Material Board, 28
Deglycerolized red blood cells, 40, 52, 98, 102–103, 145–146, 168
Department of Homeland Security, 131
Deployable Medical Systems, 81
DEPMEDS. *See* Deployable Medical Systems
Derivative unit identification code, 148
Deuter, Danny, 156
Dewitt Army Community Hospital, 30, 120
Dilworth, Semone, 191
DoD. *See* US Department of Defense

Donor History Questionnaire, 170–172
Donor recruitment campaign, 126–129
"Don't Ask, Don't Tell" policy, 170
Drew, Dr. Charles, 2
DUIC, *See* derivative unit identification code
Duncan, Vincent, 191
Dunn, Sheryl, 111

E

"Eight-Hour Hold," 83, 84
Eisenhower, Dwight, 30
Elder, Kathleen, 111, 123, 124, 126, 173, 217
ELISA. *See* Enzyme-linked immunosorbent assay
Enterprise Blood Management System, 171
Enzyme-linked immunosorbent assay, 85
Espiritu, Maria, 157
Etter, Hal, 60
Europe
    blood support units, 182–186
    European Command, 94, 97
    European Theater of Operations blood distribution during World War II, 4
    US Army blood bank, 2, 180, 182
Evans, Christopher, 133, 149, 157, 158, 192
"Exercise Nifty Nugget," 58

F

Farah, Maria, 158
FDA. *See* Food and Drug Administration
Federal Civil Defense Administration, 9
Federal Food, Drug, and Cosmetic Act, 61, 106
Feltz, Larry, 185, 186
Fenwal Laboratories, 11, 84
Fenwal Plastic blood collection bag, 11, 12
Ferguson, Specialist 4th Class, 40
Fieldman, Lieutenant Commander, 97
Fipps, Don, 188
Fitzpatrick, G. Michael, 94, 125–126, 132, 159, 204
Fitzsimons Army Medical Center, 100
Flintjer, John, 182
Food and Drug Administration
    blood donor guidelines, 125, 128
    blood industry regulation, 25
    information management requirements, 123–125, 128

licensure of blood donor centers, 59–62, 82–84, 100–101
quality assurance requirements, 105–106, 110–111, 123–124
testing requirements, 106–107, 129–130
Forward Operating Base Edinburgh, 150
406th Medical Laboratory, 30–31, 32, 36–37, 39–41
Franks, Tommy, 136
Freeze-dried plasma, 2, 5, 177
Frozen plasma, 144, 151
Frozen red blood cells, 37, 40, 52, 96–98, 102–103, 168
Frozen whole blood, 81, 96, 110, 136–137
Fryar, Ronny A., 132, 149, 166, 168, 170, 171, 175, vii–viii
Ft Belvoir, Virginia, 120
Ft Benning, Georgia, 118, 121, 166, 174, 175
Ft Bliss, Texas, 174
Ft Bragg, North Carolina, 174, 175
Ft Dix, New Jersey, 32, 34
Ft Gordon, Georgia, 174, 176
Ft Hood, Texas, 34, 58–59, 81–82, 116–118, 121
Ft Knox, Kentucky, 118, 206
Ft Leonard Wood, Missouri, 34, 138
Ft Ord, California, 77, 99
Ft Sam Houston, Texas, 34, 35

G

Gallo, Dr. Robert, 85
Gates, Robert, 136, 138–139, 144, 158
Gen-Probe, 109, 129
General Leonard Wood Army Community Hospital, 138
George Washington University, 201, 204
Golden Hour Container, 143–144
Goldwater-Nichols Department of Defense Reorganization Act of 1986, 78
Gonzales, Richard, 145, 147, 156, 171, 172, 174, 176, 189
Gottlieb, A. Matthew, 34–35, 213
Gourdine, Emmett, 118, 122–123, 140, 141
Griffin, Gary, 77
Group O blood, 32, 34, 78, 81, 102, 177
Guidelines for Quality Assurance in Blood Establishments, 106

Gulf of Tonkin Resolution, 30
Guy, Francis, 39, 40
Guzman, Juan, 192

H

Ha, Miss, 40
Haemonetics, 147
Hann, Dr. William, 202
Hannagan, Michael, 57
Hanson, Ralph, 60
Harris, April, 191
Harshbarger, Marta, 173
Hathaway, Tom, 185, 203
Hatten, John, 185
Hawley, Paul, 2–3
HCLL Transfusion, 120, 172–173
Health Affairs, 103–104
Health Care Systems Support Agency, 86
Health Facilities Planning Agency, 174, 187
Health Information Technology for Economic and Clinical Health Act, 173
Health Insurance Portability and Accountability Act of 1996, 173
Health Resource Advisory Committee, 9
Health Service Support, AirLand Battle, 81
Health Services Command, 57–60, 62, 86, 93, 100, 114–115, 221
HemCon bandage, 144
Hemorrhage control, 139–141
Hemostatic bandages, 144
Hepatitis
disease testing, 84, 105, 107, 144
World War II cases, 5
Hepatitis-associated antibody, 55, 56
Hepatitis B core antibody, 84
Hill, Ronnie, 147, 157, 192
HIV. *See* Human immunodeficiency virus
Ho Chi Minh, 30
Horoho, Patricia, 171
HSC. *See* Health Services Command
Huang, Chih, 191
Human immunodeficiency virus, 85, 106–107, 109, 129
Human T-cell lymphotropic virus, 85–87, 107–108

I

IND. *See* Investigational new drug protocol
Infectious disease testing, 84–87, 169, 173–174, 225–226
Information assurance, 172–173
Information technology, 110–111, 159–161, 172–173
International Council for Commonality in Blood Banking Automation, 124
International Society for Blood Transfusion labeling software, 123–124, 167
Interorganizational Task Force on Domestic Disasters and Acts of Terrorism, 132
Investigational new drug protocol, 129
Ismail, Sam, 157
ISU 96RC, 136
Ives, John, 107

J

Jablonski, Specialist 4th Class, 40
Jacobs, Gerald, 58, 60, 85–86
Jefferson Cup, 204
Johnson, Maria, 139, 158
Johnson, Lyndon, 30
Joint blood distribution system, 102
Joint Blood Program Office, 97, 159
Joint Blood Program officers, 156
Jordan, France F., 78

K

Kagawa, Gary, 108, 109, 129
Kahn test, 26
Kellar, Gerald, 192
Kendrick, Douglas B., 2, 29, 211
Kendrick Memorial Blood Center, 174, 176
Kennedy, John, 30
Kiel, Frank, 40
Kim Il Sung, 5
Knodel, Stewart "Stu," 81
Kontron Automation system, 186
Korean War
 Army Blood Program efforts, 5–12
 blood support units, 186–189
Krueger, Richard, 133
Kuper, Joshua, 192

L

Labeling system, 123–124
Lamoureaux, John, 176
Landstuhl, Germany, 184–186, 195–197
LaNoue, Alcide, 100
Lean Six Sigma, 122, 123
Lenn, Claude, 182
Lennette, Paul, 39, 40
Licensure, 59–62, 82–84, 93, 100–101, 114–115
Life Force recruitment theme, 126, 128
LifeTrak Donor, 120, 172–173
Lippert, Lloyd, 110
Liver testing, 84, 107
Look-back computer program, 86–87, 107
Lopatka, Mike, 120, 123
Loutit, J.F., 5
Lowery, Lionel, 157

M

Machen, Private First Class, 40
Madigan Army Medical Center, 99, 120, 122
Malloy, Wilbur, 94, 185, 187
Mann, Paul, 156
Martin, Peter, 157
Martinez, Anselmo "Papo," 107
Mascarinas, Aaron, 158
Matthews, Specialist 5th Class, 40
Mayer, Dr. William, 78
MBP. *See* Military Blood Program
MBPA. *See* Military Blood Program Agency
MBPO. *See* Military Blood Program Office
McDaniel, Steven, 157, 191
McDonald, Harry, Jr., 192
McFadden, Gwendolyn, 157
McGuire Air Force Base, 32, 34, 35
McKinley, Loran, 37
MCS9000, 141–142, 147, 168
MEDCOM. *See* US Army Medical Command
MEDCOM Mobilization Branch, 148
MEDEVAC. *See* Medical evacuation missions
Medical detachment, blood support, 189–190
Medical evacuation missions, 150–151
Medical Field Service School, 2, 35
Medical Force 2000, 81, 188–189
Medical Readiness Directorate, 78

INDEX

Medical Readiness Strategic Plan, 78, 80, 81, 102–105
Medical Reengineering Initiative, 189–190
Medical Service Corps, 182
Medical Service-Medical, Dental, and Veterinary Care, 28–29
Medical support units, 134–135, 137–139
Medical Unit Self-contained Transportable, 81
Mediware Information Systems, 120, 172
Mermite canisters, 3, 6
Messenger, Jacquelyn, 158, 192
Mester, Craig, 157, 191
Micronics, Incorporated, 145
Military Blood Program, 40–41, 48–49
Military Blood Program 2004, 78, 81
Military Blood Program Agency, 27–28, 31–32, 38, 55, 222
Military Blood Program Office, 55, 75, 78–79, 89–91
Military Field Medical Systems Standardization Steering Group, 78
Military occupational specialties, 148–149
Miller, Lieutenant Colonel Dave, 99, 111
Minnesota Thermal Science, 144
Mobile platelet collection system, 141–142, 147
Modified Table of Organization and Equipment units, 182
Mollison, P.L., 5
Mologne, Lewis, 75, 77, 186–187
Morrison, Elaine, 158, 191
MOS. *See* Military occupational specialties
MRSP. *See* Medical Readiness Strategic Plan
MSUs. *See* Medical support units
Mullins, Admiral, 170
Multinational Force-Iraq laboratory and blood officers, 156
MUST. *See* Medical Unit Self-contained Transportable

N

National Blood Donor Month, 51, 53
National Blood Donor Services, 2
National Blood Policy, 52
National Blood Program, 9, 11, 20–22
National Defense Authorization Acts, 81, 131
National Emergency Blood Program, 9, 11, 23
National Institutes of Health, 56
National Naval Medical Center, 120
National Response Plan, 132
Naval Emergency Cargo Air Delivery Systems, 187
Neel, Spurgeon, 57
9th Medical Lab, 35–36
Nixon, Richard, 51–54
Norris, Gary, 76, 117, 118, 122, 126, 137, 187
Nucleic acid testing, 109, 129
Nutricel, 82, 84

O

Obama, Barack, 149–150, 170
Ochoa, Gloria, 86, 107
Office of Defense Mobilization, 9
Office of Homeland Security, 131
Office of The Surgeon General, 2, 27, 28, 57–59, 93, 100
Operation Enduring Freedom
    Army Blood Program initiatives, 141–147
    blood product shipments, 151
    blood requirements for US Central Command, 133–135
    blood supply units and platoon leaders, 157–158
    expansion of supported hospitals, 147–149
    improving hemorrhage control on the battlefield, 139–141
    Joint Blood Program officers, 156
    proposed new blood product planning factors, 160
    reserve component support, 137–139
    units of blood transfused, 152, 154–155
Operation Iraqi Freedom
    Army Blood Program initiatives, 141–147
    blood product shipments, 151
    blood requirements for US Central Command, 135–137
    blood supply units and platoon leaders, 158
    end of combat operations, 149–151
    expansion of supported hospitals, 147–149
    improving hemorrhage control on the battlefield, 139–141
    information technology, 159–161
    Joint Blood Program officers, 156

Multinational Force-Iraq laboratory and blood officers, 156
proposed new blood product planning factors, 160
reserve component support, 137–139
units of blood transfused, 153–155
Operation New Dawn, 149–151, 155
Operation United Assistance, 190
Operations Desert Shield/Desert Storm, 94–99
Optisol, 82
OraQuick HCV rapid test, 144
Ortiz, Veronica, 191
O'Shaughnessy, Edward, 27, 28
OTSG. *See* Office of The Surgeon General

P

Paid donors, 29, 51–52
Panetta, Leon, 150, 170
Patton, George S., IV, 50, 55
Peake, James, 95
Pell, Ken, 126
Pentagon, 85, 130–131
Perry, Elaine, 130, 187, 218–219
Peterson, Herman, 133, 156
Pick, Robert, 93
PIPA. *See* Pyruvate, inosine, phosphate, and adenine solution
Pitney Bowes, 123
Platelet concentrate, 52, 82
Plateletpheresis, 140–142, 147, 168, 190
Platte, Richard, 58, 61, 77, 81, 86, 93–96, 100, 186, 203, 216
Polk, Anthony, 35, 39, 78–80, 104, 185, 214–215
Portnoy, Dr. J., 26
Powell, Colin, 134
Presidential Reserve Call-up Authority, 138–139
Procleix HIV-1/HCV assay, 129
Public Health Service, 56
Public Health Service Act, 61
Pyruvate, inosine, phosphate, and adenine solution, 96

Q

Quality assurance programs, 105–111, 122–124
Quesada, Jose, 122, 157, 191
Quesada, Major Jose, 157
QuikClot, 144

R

Radcliffe, John, 52, 57
Randall, Paul, 149, 158
Ranger Group O Low Titer Fresh Whole Blood Program, 177, 178
Rapid plasma reagin test, 26
Rapid transfusion transmitted disease diagnostic, 145, 176
Red blood cell shipments, 151
Red blood cell shipping containers, 141, 143–144
Reiber, David, 133, 157, 167–168, 172, 173, 191
Rentas, Frank, 82, 141, 150, 175
Rh negative blood, 102, 103–104
Rh Null, 55
Rhee, Syngman, 5
Ridge, Tom, 131
Rivera, Pablo, 191
Robertson, Oswald H., 1, 117, 119, xvi
Robertson Blood Center, 116–118, 121, 168
Rodgers, Jack, 34
Rogers-Bass, Ginger, 80
Rolland, SP4, 40
ROLO. *See* Ranger Group O Low Titer Fresh Whole Blood Program
Roosevelt, Franklin, 2
RPR. *See* Rapid plasma reagin test
Rumsfeld, Donald, 137, 138

S

Scheno, Mr., 60
Schmidt, Jeff, 81
Seoul Military Hospital, 27
September 11, 2001, 130–132
Service blood program officers, 81
Shipping box, 31, 32, 33
Single-donor testing, 109, 129
655th Medical Company, 184–186, 195–197
Skvorak, Michael, 182
Sloan, Melanie, 145, 156, 158, 177, 192
Smith, Captain Jeff, 142
SOLX, 147
Spectra Biologics, 55, 56
Spiker, James, Jr., 24, 27, 34, 52, 57–60, 78–79, 85, 94–95, 186–187, 200, 203, 214
Standardized labeling system, 123, 124
Stanton, Mike, 93, 94, 95, 110, 185, 186, 204

Stewart, Dennis, 108, 109
Sullivan, Gordon, 100
Sullivan, Eugene R., 174, 176
Sullivan Memorial Blood Center, 121, 174, 175
Summerville, Chet, 75
Supported military hospitals, 147–149
Swingholm, Matthew, 145, 147, 157, 175, 191
Sylvia, Bruce, 92, 97, 187
Syphilis assay, 26

T

Table of Distribution and Allowances, 148, 182
Tan Son Nhut Air Base, 35–36
Taylor, Audra, 156, 172, 178, 191, 219–220
Taylor, SP5, 40
TBBC. *See* The Blood Bank Center
TDAs. *See* Table of Distribution and Allowances
Team Spirit exercise, 187
Tejada, Luis, 191
Telemedicine and Advanced Technology Research Center, 159
Terrorism, 130–132
Terry, Teresa, 158, 192
The Blood Bank Center, 58–59
Theater Army Medical Management Information System, 99
Theater Defense Blood Standard System, 159, 161
Theater Medical Data Store-Blood, 160, 177
Thompson, Shane, 136, 158
Thompson, Specialist 4th Class, 40
ThunderCat Technology, 120
Tobias, Kenneth, 183–184
Tourniquets, 144
TRADOC. *See* Training and Doctrine Command
Training and Doctrine Command, 96, 138
Transfusion service, 29
Transfuso-Vac bottle, 1
Transmissible Spongiform Encephalopathy Advisory Committee, 125, 127, 128
Trevino, Javier, 150, 157, 191
Tripler Army Medical Center, 96, 130
Troha, Private 1st Class, 41
Truman, Harry, 6, 8, 9, 11
Tuggle, Joseph, 184, 186
Type O frozen plasma, 144

U

UD. *See* Universal donors
Ulchi Focus Lens exercise, 187
UN Monitoring, Verification, and Inspection Commission, 134
United Nations Security Council, 134
Universal donor, 34
US Africa Command, 190
US Army Blood Bank Fellowship, 27, 34, 201–210
US Army Europe Blood Bank, 180, 182
US Army Europe Blood Donor Center, 107, 108
US Army Health Services Command, 57
US Army Medical Command, 100, 123, 139, 148
US Army Medical Command Europe, 182–184
US Army Medical Field Service School, 2
US Army Medical Research Laboratory, 34, 59, 202–203, 205
US Army Medical Service Field Activities, 28
US Army Republic of Vietnam Central Blood Bank, 35–36
US Army Training and Doctrine Command, 96
US Army Vietnam Central Blood Bank, 32
US Army Western Command, 96
US Central Command, 94, 97, 133–137
US Department of Defense
    agreement with FDA for voluntary licensure of military blood banks, 61, 71–73
    Armed Forces Blood Donor Program, 6–9, 10, 14–22
    Military Blood Program Agency establishment, 27–28, 43–47
    Military Blood Program Office establishment, 55, 64–70
    operational procedures for military blood donor centers, 25
US Department of Health, Education and Welfare, 52
US Military Academy, 74, 76–77
US Transportation Command, 79
Usry, Robert, 58, 60

V

Vampire Program, 150–151
Van Ronzelen, Debbie, 173
VDRL. *See* Venereal disease research laboratory test

Venereal disease research laboratory test, 27
Vietnam War
    Army Blood Program efforts, 30–41
    post-war Army Blood Program efforts, 51–57
Virchis, Hiram, 191
Voluntary blood donation, 40–41, 48–49, 52, 54

W

Walden, William, 138
Walson Air Force Hospital, 93
Walson Army Hospital, 34
Walter Reed Army Institute of Research, 29, 205
Walter Reed Army Medical Center, 28–30, 52, 57, 61, 77, 120, 206–209
Walter Reed General Hospital, 2
Walter Reed National Military Medical Center, 120, 210
Ward, Mike, 78, 79, 80
Watt, James E., 182
Webster, Noel, 103, 109, 122, 123, 141, 156, 187, 188, 217218
Weinberger, Casper, 52
West Nile virus, 129–130, 173

West Point Military Academy, 74, 76–77
Western Star, 85–86
Whitacre, Robin, 120, 122, 136, 156
Whittaker, Donna, 100, 122, 123, 126, 219
Whole blood pathogen reduction device, 147, 176
Whole Blood Program, 40–41, 48–49
William Beaumont Army Medical Center, 174
Williams, SP5, 40
Wilson, Charles E., 9
Wilson, Jason, 60
Winkler, Bill, 78
Winkler, Sergeant First Class Phil, 80
Woods, Woody, 78, 79
World War II
    Army Blood Program efforts, 1–5
WRAMC. *See* Walter Reed Army Medical Center
Wrenn, Major Hubert, 60

Z

Z-Medica, 144
Zielmanski, Ken, 81, 96
Zika virus, 173